Dr. Miriam Stoppard

NATURAL
MENOPAUSE

HEALTHCARE

DK PUBLISHING, I

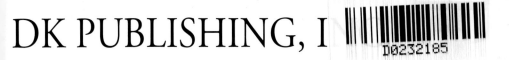

A DK PUBLISHING BOOK

DESIGN AND EDITORIAL   Kelly Flynn Associates

SENIOR MANAGING ART EDITOR   Lynne Brown
MANAGING EDITOR   Jemima Dunne

SENIOR ART EDITOR   Karen Ward
SENIOR EDITOR   Penny Warren
US EDITORS   Jill Hamilton, Iris Rosoff

PRODUCTION   Antony Heller

First American Edition, 1998
4 6 8 10 9 7 5 3
Published in the United States by
DK Publishing, Inc. , 95 Madison Avenue
New York, New York 10016

www.dk.com

Material in this publication was previously published by DK Publishing, Inc.
in *Menopause* by Dr. Miriam Stoppard.

Library of Congress Cataloging-in-Publication Data
Stoppard, Miriam.
    Natural menopause / by Miriam Stoppard. -- 1st American ed.
    p.   cm. -- (DK healthcare series)
    Includes index.
    ISBN 0-7894-3090-8
    1. Menopause--Popular works. 2. Naturopathy--Popular works.
I. Title. II. Series
RG186.S763 1998
612.6'65--dc21
                                                        97-48453
                                                           CIP

Reproduced by Colourscan, Singapore and IGS, Radstock, Avon
Printed in Hong Kong by Wing King Tong

CONTENTS

INTRODUCTION 6

CHAPTER 1

WHAT HAPPENS AT MENOPAUSE 7

PLANNING YOUR FUTURE 8
THE RANGE OF SYMPTOMS 10

CHAPTER 4

PHYSICAL HEALTH 47

GOOD NUTRITION • WEIGHT CONTROL
• KEEPING FIT • ABANDONING BAD HABITS
• CARING FOR YOUR BODY

CHAPTER 2

MENOPAUSAL MEDICAL COMPLAINTS 27

OSTEOPOROSIS • HEART ATTACKS AND STROKES
• UROGENITAL AGING • BREAST CANCER

CHAPTER 5

NATURAL THERAPIES 71

NATUROPATHY • AROMATHERAPY • HOMEOPATHY
• HERBALISM • ACUPUNCTURE • ACUPRESSURE
• HYDROTHERAPY • MASSAGE • OSTEOPATHY
• CHIROPRACTIC • YOGA

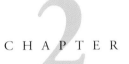

CHAPTER 3

POSITIVE ATTITUDES 35

THINKING POSITIVELY 36
CHANGING FAMILY ROLES 38
MENTAL AGILITY 40
RELAXATION 42
YOUR APPEARANCE 44

CHAPTER 6

SEXUALITY AND RELATIONSHIPS 81

NATURAL SATISFACTION 82
MAXIMIZE LOVEMAKING 86
BIRTH CONTROL 90
POSTMENOPAUSAL RELATIONSHIPS 92

INDEX 94 • ACKNOWLEDGMENTS 96

INTRODUCTION

FOR MANY WOMEN, menopause can be a psychological, emotional, and intellectual turning point in their lives as well as a physical one, but it does not have to mean a decline. As your children leave home and you look forward to reducing your workload, you will have more time to yourself than you have ever had before. This can be liberating, and you can take the opportunity to reassess your lifestyle and make decisions about what you want from the future.

As menopause approaches, the ovaries begin to fail, and there is a sudden dip in our female sex hormones, estrogen and progesterone, which causes the cessation of menstruation. About three-quarters of all women experience some menopausal symptoms, all of which can be treated.

Temporary symptoms of menopause include hot flashes, night sweats, and loss of libido, and they may last for several years; long-term ones include thinning and drying out of vaginal and genital skin and urinary troubles – all of which may become permanent. Fortunately, these complaints are not dangerous and can be remedied by many therapies. However, some of the other consequences of menopause *are* dangerous. One of these is osteoporosis or brittle bones, and one in four postmenopausal women who is admitted to the hospital with a fractured femur never returns home, so it is important that we protect ourselves from this disease.

Menopause affects every organ of a woman's body, and any treatment, therefore, must be viewed in the context of what is good for the whole: this involves a healthy diet, lots of regular exercise, relaxation, yoga, minerals, and whatever change in your lifestyle you think would help. Each of the complementary therapies, from aromatherapy to yoga, for instance, has its own advocates.

CHAPTER

1

WHAT HAPPENS AT MENOPAUSE

As the supply of eggs in the ovaries dwindles, estrogen and progesterone levels fluctuate and begin to decline. This results in the end of menstruation and also has other effects on the body. Menopausal symptoms are felt largely because of the suddenness of estrogen withdrawal. Many women experience few or no symptoms while others may be incapacitated. This chapter describes the classic symptoms associated with menopause and gives self-help advice plus the most appropriate natural therapy available.

PLANNING YOUR FUTURE

Menopause is an important crossroads in our lives that, if viewed positively, can be both rewarding and revealing. Life is a series of milestones and, where in our younger days we rushed past the markers, as we grow older, we tend to reflect more. Menopause gives us a perfect opportunity to look back at what we have already done in the past and decide what we might want to do in the future.

A woman who may have devoted half of her life to raising a family still has time to go back to college, start a new career, and take care of her body so that she is fitter than she has ever been. The end of fertility doesn't have to imply new restrictions and physical decline; our options can increase rather than decrease.

MENOPAUSE TIMETABLE

We often use the word menopause incorrectly. Strictly speaking, it means the end of menstruation and it could, hypothetically, be a moment in time. The word "climacteric" more accurately describes the ongoing changes and symptoms, since it refers to a transition period that may last 15–20 years. During this phase, both ovarian function and hormonal production decline, and the body adjusts itself to these changes.

It may help to think of menopause as being the counterpart of menarche, when menstrual periods commence. The climacteric can then be compared with the years of adolescence, or puberty, when the ovaries begin to function and mature.

THE CLIMACTERIC

There are three stages in the climacteric: pre-, peri-, and postmenopause. Menopause signals the end of the premenopause and the beginning of the postmenopause.

Premenopause This period of time refers to the early years of the climacteric, after the age of 40, when menstrual periods may become irregular and sometimes heavy, and the symptoms of menopause start to emerge. You find yourself saying, "Is it hot in here or just me?" If your doctor tells you that you are premenopausal, ask for a precise definition of what he or she means.

Perimenopause This is the stage lasting several years on either side of your last menstrual period. Perimenopause is, in part, a retrospective diagnosis, since it's only when your periods cease that you can measure backward two years in time to when it began. It's during this time that you notice most physical changes, when your periods may become irregular, and when hot flashes may start.

Menopause This has a precise meaning – menopause is your final menstrual period. This is another date that can only be identified retrospectively, when you have not had menstrual bleeding for 12 months. In other words, it is impossible for a woman to know the exact moment that she is experiencing menopause.

Postmenopause This period overlaps with the end of the perimenopausal stage and will extend into the years that follow your last menstrual period. It lasts until the end of your life.

CAN I PREDICT MY LAST PERIOD?

The average age when women experience menopause in this country is 51, an age that has remained fairly constant over the centuries, even though the average age for the onset of menstruation has become earlier. About half of all women will stop menstruating before they turn 51 and half will stop menstruating afterward. There is no need to be alarmed if you stop menstruating before your 45th birthday; this happens to about a third of all women. At the other end of the scale, many women continue menstruating into their early 50s, and a few into their mid-50s.

Although there is no way in which you can predict exactly when menopause will occur, there are factors that may influence its timing. The age you begin to menstruate may affect the age that you experience menopause, although no studies have yet proved this. And it is possible that the age at which your mother experienced menopause will have some bearing on when you stop menstruating, but again, this relationship has not been scientifically proven. Two factors that do *not* influence the time of menopause are whether or not you used oral contraceptives and the age at which you had your first and last children.

THE RANGE OF SYMPTOMS

The list of symptoms associated with menopause is long, and at first glance may be daunting. Fortunately, no woman experiences the whole range – you will probably have only a few of the symptoms and many women have none. The list described here is long simply because it's helpful to know the array of disparate symptoms, especially if you need to discuss your treatment with a doctor. The physical effects of menopause are so diverse, it is sometimes hard to connect them to a single cause. There are some classic symptoms, such as hot flashes and mood swings, that women may readily associate with menopause, but others, such as poor bladder control or back pain, often appear to be just incidental. All the symptoms listed here are directly or indirectly related to a drop in estrogen levels.

Back pain
Breast soreness
Chest pain
Itchy skin
Night sweats
Palpitations

Anxiety and low self-esteem
Depressed mood
Dry hair, eyes, and mouth,
and dry, wrinkled skin
Feelings of pessimism
Forgetfulness
Headaches
Hot flashes
Inability to concentrate or
make decisions
Increase in facial hair
Insomnia
Irritability and tearfulness
Lowering of the voice
Mood swings and PMS
Thin hair
Fatigue and lethargy

Aches and pains
Brittle nails
Muscle soreness
Pins and needles
Swollen or stiff joints

Bloated abdomen
Constipation
Dry vagina
Heavy/irregular periods
Itchy vulva
Loss of bladder control
Loss of libido
Slower sexual arousal and
lubrication
Urgent urination

Signs of menopause

The early symptoms associated with menopause, such as mood swings, are different from later symptoms, which include dry skin and slower sexual arousal. This reflects the body's response to fluctuating estrogen levels, and then to permanently lowered estrogen levels.

HOT FLASHES

Hot flashes are experienced by more than 85 percent of menopausal women, although both their frequency and severity can vary greatly from person to person. During a hot flash, a woman can perspire so profusely that perspiration runs down her face, neck, and back; her skin will become hot, her heart will beat faster, and she may well also experience palpitations. In rare cases, a woman may actually faint during a hot flash.

Hot flashes occur because the brain decides that the body is overheated. We now know that this is because the natural temperature set-point (the temperature above which the brain considers the body too hot and below which it considers it too cold) is lowered. This means that even under normal conditions the brain may think that the body's temperature is too high, and responds by increasing the blood flow through the skin to reduce it. The skin then reddens and begins to perspire, and when the sweat starts to evaporate, the body temperature cools down again. Even though a hot flash may feel most severe in the head, face, and neck, the rise in temperature actually occurs throughout the body. Finger and toe temperatures also rise sharply at the beginning of a hot flash.

In a Danish study of menopausal women, one third of those interviewed continued to have hot flashes for ten years after their last period, and in the most severe cases, women had hot flashes six or seven times every hour. Two out of every three women suffered hot flashes well before their last menstrual period, but for most, the frequency increased dramatically at menopause and continued for about the next five or six years.

The discomfort experienced during a hot flash is unique – it is not, for example, the same as being overheated. In one study, investigators tried to induce hot flashes by using hot-water bottles and blankets, but they discovered that applying direct external heat does not produce the same dramatic changes in heart rate and blood pressure that a menopausal hot flash does.

HOT FLASHES SELF-HELP

The following simple measures can relieve symptoms.

- *Record your flashes; try to avoid situations that seem to act as a trigger.*

- *Don't wear synthetic fabrics, and avoid clothes with high necks and long sleeves.*

- *Discover ways of cooling down: keep a thermos of ice water near you, take a cold shower, or use a fan.*

- *Give up smoking.*

- *Try taking vitamin E. One thousand IUs a day is recommended. Avoid vitamin E if you suffer from diabetes or heart problems.*

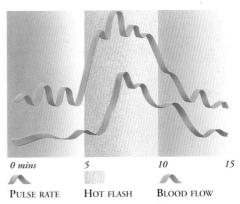

| 0 mins | 5 | 10 | 15 |

PULSE RATE   HOT FLASH   BLOOD FLOW

Hot flash sensation
Before you experience a flash, your blood flow (see above) increases dramatically and your pulse rate becomes faster. Flashes usually last for about three to five minutes.

NIGHT SWEATS SELF-HELP

The following simple measures can relieve symptoms.

• *Keep your bedroom temperature fairly cool, and leave a window open if possible.*

• *Avoid nightgowns and bed-clothes made of nylon or polyester; cotton fabrics will be more comfortable.*

• *Keep a bowl of tepid water and a sponge by your bed so that you can cool yourself down easily. Never use cold water since it can cause you to become overheated. Allow the water to evaporate on your skin – as it does so it will take the heat and make you feel cooler.*

COMPLEMENTARY THERAPY

The products that are most frequently suggested by herbalists and homeopaths for hot flashes are lachesis, fo-ti-tieng, pulsatilla, white willow, wild yam root, dong quai, soybeans, black cohosh, and sage. You can find all of them in most healthfood stores and at pharmacies that stock natural products. Alternatively, you can consult a qualified homeopath or herbalist.

Sage, dong quai, and black cohosh contain estrogen-like substances. It is the mild estrogenic effect they exert on the body that may help compensate for declining levels of natural hormone.

Acupuncture can relieve hot flashes. Both electro-stimulated acupuncture (ESA) and superficial needles position acupuncture (SNPA) decreased the number of flashes by almost half in a sample of menopausal women in Stockholm. This change persisted for three months after the treatment.

DIET AND EXERCISE

Limiting your intake of foods and drinks that trigger hot flashes can help reduce their intensity. These include sugary, salty, spicy, or hot dishes, chocolate, alcohol, coffee, tea, and cola drinks. Avoid large meals (small, regular ones are better) and include soy-based products, such as soy sauce and tofu, and citrus fruits – all of which have estrogenic properties – in your diet. Regular exercise helps too; women who exercise regularly have fewer hot flashes than those who do not.

NIGHT SWEATS

The nighttime equivalent of the hot flash is the night sweat, in which you wake up hot and drenched in perspiration. Most women who experience night sweats also have hot flashes during the daytime, but the reverse isn't always so. Night sweats can occasionally be a symptom of stress, or even a disease that is unrelated to menopause. If you consult your doctor, he or she will be able to make a diagnosis.

Sleeplessness in menopausal women is nearly always linked to night sweats. Sufferers describe waking up, so drenched in perspiration that they have to get up to change their nightgowns and sheets.

We know from research that night sweat is a physiological process involving a fever that lasts a minute or two and then disappears. The heart rhythm goes wild, the body temperature rises, and the woman is left with a sweaty face and chest, followed by a feeling of being chilled. Some women with severe and frequent night sweats become very depressed. Their depression doesn't usually go away until the night sweats are brought under control.

COMPLEMENTARY THERAPY

There are several herbal remedies that may alleviate insomnia. Scullcap, for instance, is generally regarded as a good sedative herb, and can be combined with lemon balm to treat anxiety that leads to insomnia. Camomile and sage also have soothing properties and make refreshing and effective herbal teas. Sage tea has a particularly strong taste, but if it is not to your liking, you can buy sage in tablet form from any good herbalist. Agnus castus is an excellent general herb for many menopausal symptoms including both hot flashes and night sweats. Since it may help normalize female hormone levels, it acts as a natural type of hormone replacement therapy.

Relaxation can be particularly therapeutic because it calms the mind and body, which in turn normalizes body chemistry and makes the skin sweat less. Meditation can be useful too. It slows down your metabolism. It can slow down your brain waves from the fast beta waves that are characteristic of the normal working day to a slower alpha or theta wave, the wave pattern that occurs just before sleeping. If you can achieve this state, it can be as restful as sleep. See pp. 42–43 for a selection of simple but effective relaxation and meditation techniques. Or try yoga, which can have a calming effect. See p. 80 for some easy-to-practice techniques.

DIET AND EXERCISE

Avoiding the types of food and drink listed on p. 12 can help alleviate the frequency and intensity of night sweats as well as hot flashes. In addition, try to avoid eating large meals late in the evening if you suffer from night sweats. If possible, eat your main meal during the day at lunchtime and have only a light supper during the early part of the evening.

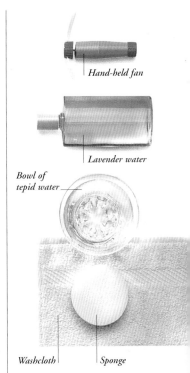

Hand-held fan

Lavender water

Bowl of tepid water

Washcloth *Sponge*

Relief from night sweats
Cooling yourself with tepid water will help ease the discomfort of night sweats. A battery-operated fan and scented lavender water can also be efficient cooling aids.

VAGINAL AND URINARY SYMPTOMS

Urogenital problems are particularly common during menopause, yet only four in ten women consult their doctor about them. Anatomically, the vagina and the lower urinary tract lie very close to each other, separated by just a few layers of cells. They both decline when there is a lack of estrogen by becoming thin and dry.

Urinary symptoms include discomfort in urinating and frequent and urgent urination, even when there is very little liquid in the bladder. There may also be some dribbling because the sphincter muscle guarding the exit from the bladder becomes weaker due to low estrogen levels. From time to time, urine escapes from the bladder when one laughs, coughs, or carries a heavy weight. This is called stress incontinence and is due to increased pressure inside the abdomen squeezing urine from the bladder. With many of these symptoms, you could also have genital dryness and itching. Vaginal soreness, particularly during or after intercourse because the vagina fails to lubricate, is also very common among menopausal and postmenopausal women.

COMPLEMENTARY THERAPY

Herbs that may relieve urinary symptoms include buchu, cornsilk, and uva-ursi, which has some antiseptic properties. Goldenseal is believed to have some anti-infective properties.

DIET AND EXERCISE

Keep your bladder flushed out by drinking at least four pints (two liters) of fluid a day – water is best. Try cranberry juice too; this is especially effective if you are prone to cystitis. Exercise can also help keep your vaginal area supple. Swimming is a particularly good exercise, but so is regular sex or masturbation.

Kegel exercises strengthen pelvic muscles, combat urinary incontinence, and make sex more pleasurable, and they are simple to do. To find out which muscles to exercise, next time you go to the bathroom stop urinating in midstream by contracting your muscles; these are your pelvic floor muscles. Using these muscles, draw them up, hold for a count of five, then relax. Repeat this five times and do at least ten times a day.

MUSCLE AND JOINT SYMPTOMS

Collagen is a protein that provides the scaffolding for every tissue in the body, and when it begins to disintegrate at menopause, muscles lose their bulk, strength, and coordination, and joints become stiff. Muscles are more prone to soreness and stiffness after exercise, and joints may swell so that their mobility becomes restricted. If you retain fluid, you may get pins and needles or numbness in the hands.

Osteoporosis (often called the brittle bones disease) causes aches and pains all over the body, especially in the upper back due to the thinning of vertebrae.

General fatigue during menopause may be profound. Although underused muscles and joints can be a major factor in this, there are other causes of chronic fatigue that do not necessarily have any direct connection with menopause, such as low blood sugar, anemia, and an underactive thyroid gland. Make sure you have your doctor check out all of these possibilities if you are experiencing disabling fatigue.

COMPLEMENTARY THERAPY

If you are suffering from stiff and swollen joints, a poultice made with cayenne pepper may be helpful. Other herbal remedies that could be effective include alfalfa, sarsaparilla, feverfew, and white willow. Juniper, rosemary, and lavender essential oils may relieve pain when they are diluted with a base oil and used in a local massage or compress (see p. 73). Basil diluted with a base oil may alleviate fatigue.

DIET AND EXERCISE

Diet can help protect your muscles, bones, and joints, and, in particular, a diet containing increased amounts of calcium: dairy foods are high in calcium (cheeses such as Parmesan and cheddar are particularly good), as are oily fish, such as sardines and anchovies, and soy-based products, such as soy sauce and tofu. If you don't feel that you can increase your calcium-rich food intake easily, ask your doctor to recommend a good calcium supplement. In addition to a calcium-rich diet, weight-bearing exercises, such as skipping, brisk walking, and dancing, are known to help strengthen bones.

MUSCLE AND JOINT SELF-HELP

Try to exercise regularly. If you keep your muscles strong with exercise, you will be more agile and, if you do fall, muscle strength and coordination will help you fall with less impact.

PREMENSTRUAL SYNDROME

If you have suffered from premenstrual syndrome (PMS) all your life, you are more likely to experience intensified symptoms, such as fatigue, anxiety, irritability, tearfulness, breast soreness, water retention, skin problems, and insomnia, as you become menopausal. If you suspect that your mood swings are PMS-related, you can confirm it by charting your symptoms daily for three months.

COMPLEMENTARY THERAPY

The standard remedy for PMS is evening primrose oil, which is widely available at health-food stores and most pharmacies. Other herbs that may be useful include bethroot, which can help alleviate very heavy or irregular periods, and black cohosh. Aromatherapists recommend the oils of ylang-ylang, lavender, and lemongrass, which you can use in a warm bath.

DIET AND EXERCISE

Premenstrual symptoms should disappear along with your periods, but while you are still menstruating there is no instant cure. You can lessen the problem, however, if you try to avoid stressful situations and eat a regular,

CHANGES DUE TO COLLAGEN DEFICIENCY

Skin	Dryness or oiliness, wrinkles, flaking, bruise easily, wounds heal slowly, patches of brown pigmentation, prominent veins
Nails	Brittleness, white spots, splinter hemorrhages appear
Eyes	Dryness, dark circles under eyes, small yellow lumps of fat on the white part of the eyes, night vision deteriorates, red blood vessels around the corners of the eyes
Gums	Bleeding and sponginess, recession leaving tooth roots exposed, infection and periodontal disease, which causes bad breath
Hair	Dullness, dryness, oiliness, split ends, poor growth, thin patches, dermatitis of the scalp, hair loss, dandruff
Mouth	Cracks on the corners of the lips, mouth ulcers that are slow to heal
Tongue	The sides may become scalloped and the tongue thinner and smoother

balanced diet throughout the month, avoiding sugar and salt (salt increases water retention and bloating). Avoiding alcohol before your period starts could also help. Exercise can alleviate premenstrual symptoms too: it's a great mood-lifter and can help work off tension and anxiety.

FACE AND SKIN SYMPTOMS

The lowered estrogen levels that occur at menopause cause changes in skin, hair, nails, eyes, mouth, and gums. These are due in part to the disintegration of collagen fibers and the weakening of the protein elastin, which gives connective tissue its strength and suppleness. One of the most noticeable changes is the appearance of wrinkles in the facial skin. Deterioration of nerve endings in the aging skin can lead to itchiness and a condition called formication, an intense tingling that some women describe as a feeling that insects are crawling across their skin. Formication is a classic symptom of menopausal distress. In a study of 5,000 women, one in five suffered from it within 12–24 months after their last menstrual period. About one in ten women continued to suffer from formication for more than 12 years after menopause.

DIET AND EXERCISE

Make sure that you eat foods rich in vitamins A, B, C, and E in addition to potassium, zinc, magnesium, bioflavonoids, iron, and calcium (see p. 50 and p. 52 for examples of vitamin- and mineral-rich foods). Drinking four pints (two liters) of water a day will not only help keep your bladder healthy, it will also have a noticeable effect on skin and hair. Regular exercise – even a daily brisk walk in the fresh air – can also benefit your skin.

SEXUAL SYMPTOMS

A common myth about menopause is that it marks the beginning of a woman's sexual decline. Nothing could be farther from the truth. The majority of women can continue to experience sexual pleasure well into old age. Most menopausal women, however, notice some changes in the way their bodies respond during arousal and sex. This is often due to physical changes in the urogenital tract rather than a decreased emotional desire for sex. One of the most common sexual problems after

FACE AND SKIN SELF-HELP

The following simple measures can help protect your face and skin.

- *Keep your skin moisturized. Avoid soap and use cleansing lotions instead.*

- *Take special care of your nails. Give yourself a manicure and pedicure every eight weeks.*

- *Rinse mouth and tongue ulcers immediately with salty water or use a proprietary ointment.*

- *Protect your skin from the sun. Avoid direct sun at all times, and when you go out in sunny weather, wear sunblock. If possible, limit your exposure to the early and late parts of the day.*

The sexual woman
Ideally, menopause should be a time when we become more open and uninhibited about our bodies.

menopause is lack of lubrication. The vaginal lining may actually crack and bleed, and this can make penetration painful and sometimes impossible.

In youth, blood flows quickly to the genitals during arousal, causing swelling and sensitivity to touch. After menopause, however, there is much less engorgement of the clitoris, the vagina, and the vulva, leading to a more subdued arousal.

The breasts also increase in size during sexual arousal in young women – by as much as a quarter in some cases. The rush of blood to the tiny veins of the breasts that causes this does not occur as often after the level of estrogen has declined. As a result, the breasts may no longer be as sensitive to stroking. Another part of the sexual response that disappears is the "sex flush" – a rash that may appear on a woman's chest and body just before orgasm. This does not affect sexual enjoyment, but it does show that your body responds to sexual arousal differently than the way it used to.

In a young woman, the vagina expands during sexual arousal to allow easy penetration. After menopause, it does not expand as much, but still remains large enough to accommodate an erect penis (as long as you allow time to achieve proper lubrication). Sexual desire can also be diminished by certain medicines, such as tranquilizers, muscle relaxants, antidepressants, amphetamines, diuretics, antihypertensives, and hormones.

Women who have had a hysterectomy or surgical removal of the ovaries may also experience a diminished enjoyment of sex and a reduced ability to reach orgasm.

COMPLEMENTARY THERAPY

Herbs have always been used to treat low sex drive, although some, such as nutmeg, have been found to irritate the urogenital system and should be avoided. Many plants, such as ginseng and saffron crocus, are widely used for their aphrodisiac properties. The bark of an African tree, *yohimbine*, is the source of several medicines used to treat impotence.

DIET AND EXERCISE

Hypothyroidism becomes more common during menopausal years, and may be a cause of low sexual desire. Since several minerals, most importantly zinc, can help activate the thyroid gland, adding zinc-rich foods such as wheatgerm and sardines to your diet can help symptoms, as can avoiding foods such as turnips, kale, cabbage, and soybeans that contain an anti-thyroid substance. Stress, such as bereavement, moving, and family problems, can also adversely affect sex drive, while too much sugar, fat, coffee, or alcohol places a strain on the body. Practicing Kegel exercises (see p. 14) regularly will give you better-toned pelvic muscles, which will enable you to grip your partner's penis more tightly and increase your sexual enjoyment.

INSOMNIA

If you are feeling depressed or anxious, or if you are suffering badly from night sweats, it can become very difficult to get to sleep and quite common to wake early in the morning. Eventually, a good night's rest can become something of a rarity.

Women who have normal levels of estrogen fall asleep faster than women who don't and spend more time in the deepest (dream) stage of sleep. They also feel more refreshed when they wake up. Dreaming seems to be particularly important for the feeling of rest and renewal that comes from sleeping. Without estrogen, we can sleep through an entire night but still feel very tired when we wake up.

COMPLEMENTARY THERAPY

Valerian root has been used for many centuries as a sleep-inducing herb, and its sedative effect can be very therapeutic during the menopausal years. Insomnia can also be alleviated by nighttime infusions of herbs such as passion flower, catnip, camomile, and hops.

DIET AND EXERCISE

The traditional glass of warm milk at bedtime does actually work for many insomniacs (this could be due to the action of calcium on the nerves) and is always worth trying. If you can, avoid eating large, heavy meals in the evening and, in particular, eat your evening meal early, preferably before seven, and try to avoid caffeinated coffees and teas. A long walk about an hour before bedtime or some other form of aerobic exercise can also improve the quality of your sleep.

INSOMNIA SELF-HELP

The following simple measures can relieve symptoms.

• *Rid yourself of night sweats or bring them under control (see p. 12) so that you can sleep undisturbed.*

• *Read a good book, or a chapter from a good book; by getting "out" of yourself, it will help you relax, which should make it easier to go to sleep.*

STOMACH AND BOWEL SYMPTOMS

Bloating with abdominal distension may be a problem during menopause. As we age, small pockets of tissue may balloon out from the bowel, giving rise to the condition called diverticulitis. Within these small pockets (*diverticula*), food may lodge, become stale, ferment, and produce large amounts of gas. The intestine may end up coated with food remnants that form small centers of fermentation. It is quite common for the sufferer to wake in the morning with a flat stomach and for the abdomen to swell as the day progresses, so that by bedtime the swelling resembles a six-month pregnancy! During the night, lack of food and sugar in the intestine allows fermentation to abate. After a breakfast that contains sugars and yeasts, fermentation in the bowels flares up again.

Because the female hormones progesterone and estrogen affect the speed at which food moves through the intestines – progesterone reduces movement so that bowel motions become infrequent, dry, and pebblelike, while estrogen speeds them up, enabling the stools to revert to a normal consistency and frequency – constipation is another frequent menopause symptom.

COMPLEMENTARY THERAPY

There are several homeopathic and herbal remedies widely available that can relieve stomach and bowel symptoms, such as the Bach Flower Remedies. Gentle "scouring" herbs and foods, such as sunflower seeds, may help, and senna has a mild purgative action. Some people recommend colonic irrigation, in which the lower part of the intestine is flushed out with water.

DIET AND EXERCISE

The classic cures for improving stomach and bowel symptoms are nearly all diet-based. Following a high-fiber diet and drinking plenty of fluids will help keep your bowel movements normal (see p. 53 for examples of high-fiber foods). Foods that cause fermentation, such as yeast-based products and sugar, should either be avoided or eaten only in the early part of the day. And if you suffer from constipation, the best cure is still a natural one – lots of figs and prunes!

BREAST SYMPTOMS

Most women experience breast discomfort in the week before they menstruate, due to fluid retention in the breast tissue and a consequent increase in breast tension. As women reach their early 40s, this discomfort may develop into a more severe pain called mastalgia. The breasts become hard, tender, and extremely painful. An attack of mastalgia can last for up to ten days.

In severe cases, the breasts can be so painful that you cannot bear anything to touch them. Pain is especially intense in the nipples and may keep you awake at night; even turning over in bed can be agony. It is estimated that 70 percent of women in this country suffer from breast pain at some time in their lives, but particularly in the pre- and perimenopausal years.

Mastalgia can often be cyclical, fluctuating with the menstrual cycle and usually becoming worse immediately before menstruation. But noncyclical mastalgia can occur at any time of the month and is most common in women over 40 years of age. The causes are not completely understood, but mastalgia may stem from abnormal sensitivity of breast tissue to the fluctuation of female hormones during menopause.

If you are suffering from severe mastalgia, you may be frightened that the pain is due to breast cancer. In the majority of cases, mastalgia is a benign condition, but you should see your doctor or have a mammogram if you need reassurance.

COMPLEMENTARY THERAPY

One of the essential fatty acids, gamolenic acid, which is found in evening primrose oil, significantly reduces breast pain in up to 70 percent of women and has not been found to have any side effects.

DIET AND EXERCISE

A bad diet can make breast problems worse. Women who suffer from breast pain tend to have low levels of essential fatty acids and eat high levels of saturated fat; saturated fat seems to exaggerate the effects of female hormones on breast tissue. Cutting down the amount of saturated fat you eat can help relieve your symptoms; see pp. 54–55 for more information on this.

BREAST SELF-HELP

One of the simplest things you can do to help maintain breast health is to examine yourself for lumps regularly, at least once a month, by following the steps below.

• *Stand naked in front of a mirror with your arms by your sides.*

• *Now raise them and put your hands behind your head; look for differences in the shape or texture of both the breasts and nipples.*

• *Feel your breasts; lie on your back with your shoulders slightly raised.*

• *Hold your fingers flat and carefully examine each section of your breast, using gentle circular movements (use your right hand to feel your left breast and vice versa).*

• *Move your hand in a clockwise circular direction on the left breast and counterclockwise on the right; keep the arm you aren't using by your side.*

• *Complete your examination by extending the arm you are not using behind your head and checking for lumps along the collarbone and in your armpits.*

WEIGHT GAIN

Some postmenopausal women strive to maintain their premenopausal weight. Medically this is quite unsound: the weight that you may gain during menopause is due to a slower metabolism – something that affects men and women as they grow older – and a decline in estrogen levels, which affects the way that fat is distributed.

Middle-aged women who are 8–12 lb (3.5–4.5 kg) underweight do not live as long as those who are 8–12 lb (3.5–4.5 kg) overweight. I don't wish to encourage any woman to become obese, but I do wish to free her from the pressure to be thin.

DIET AND EXERCISE

Unless you are so overweight that your health is being affected, a little weight gain during menopause requires no treatment. But if your weight is posing a threat to your health, and you have other risk factors for heart disease, such as high blood pressure and smoking, then it is a good idea to make changes in your diet. It is important, however, to be realistic and to be aware that changes in body shape happen to all postmenopausal women. Excessive dieting is unhealthy, and it may mean that you fail to meet your daily calcium requirements. By eating healthy foods and exercising regularly, you should remain fit and not gain weight. If you were not overweight before menopause and are no more than 13–18 lb (6–8 kg) more after it, and if your waist-to-hip ratio is not in the high risk category, then there is no health advantage in reducing your weight.

LOWERING OF THE VOICE

There are two reasons for the voice deepening after menopause. First, there is a relative increase in the male hormones, or androgens, circulating in the blood. Long after ovaries stop secreting estrogen, they continue to secrete androgens. This relative excess of male hormones has a masculinizing effect on various organs of the body, causing a deepening of the voice.

The second cause is hypothyroidism. The voice becomes deep, gruff, and slightly hoarse, and there are other symptoms, such as hair loss, a tendency to feel the cold, and fatigue. If you are suffering from hypothyroidism, (underactive thyroid) your voice will return to normal when you start to take thyroid supplements. If you feel medical treatment is necessary, you should consult your doctor as soon as you notice that your voice is deepening.

HEART SYMPTOMS

After the menopause, heart disease becomes as common in women as it is in men. Heart problems are rare in pre-menopausal women because of the presence of estrogen. Angina, a crushing pain in the middle of the chest brought on by effort and alleviated by rest, is the warning sign. Without rest, the pain can worsen and radiate up into the neck and teeth, and down the arm. Eventually the pain will become so bad that you will be forced to stop what you are doing. Angina is the sign that insufficient oxygen is reaching your heart muscle. You should take chest pain seriously and go to your doctor for a cardiac checkup.

Other symptoms relating to heart health include palpitations and shortness of breath when you exert yourself. You may find that normal exercise leaves you unusually breathless, and climbing up several flights of stairs gives you a pumping, fluttery feeling in your chest.

If you are suffering from other symptoms, such as dizziness, headaches, or blurred vision, have your blood pressure checked because you may have hypertension.

DIET AND EXERCISE

Because obesity is a risk factor in heart disease, you should try to lose weight if you are more than a few pounds over your ideal weight (see p. 22). Cut back on saturated fats, avoid sugar and other "empty" calorie foods, and try to limit the amount of salt you eat. A diet that is high in fruits and vegetables, oily fish, and legumes, and low in animal fats and rich dairy products, can help lower your cholesterol levels and reduce the risk of heart problems. Garlic can improve your cardiovascular health too; use it in cooking or take garlic pearls, which are odorless. There is a clear, direct link between smoking and increased risk of heart disease. Therefore, one of the most effective measures any woman can take to protect her heart is to stop smoking and the earlier, the better.

Regular aerobic exercise helps strengthen a weak heart and will also help reduce high blood pressure, which can lead to heart problems. Try swimming, bicycling, and

MEDICAL TREATMENT FOR HEART SYMPTOMS

There is a wide range of medicines to treat heart conditions, including antihypertensives, betablockers, diuretics, cardiac stimulants, and coronary vasodilators.

• *Angina, for instance, can be controlled by taking a coronary vasodilator whenever you have an attack – you can even take one of these tablets before exercising to prevent angina in the first place.*

• *If you suffer from high cholesterol, your doctor will probably prescribe medication to lower it to reduce the possibility of serious heart complications, and will recommend that you alter your diet (see left).*

• *If you develop heart disease, treatments available include an artificial pacemaker, a coronary bypass operation, or balloon angioplasty, depending on the type of heart condition you have.*

Body shape and heart disease
Before menopause, the waist-to-hip ratio is less than 0.8 and there is a correspondingly low risk of heart disease. After menopause, fat distribution changes and the risk of heart disease increases. You can assess your risk by dividing your waist measurement by your hip measurement. If the resulting figure is over 0.8 you fall into a higher risk group for heart disease.
For example:
32 ÷ 39 in = 0.74 (low risk)
29 ÷ 39 in = 0.81 (higher risk)

KEY

▓▓ WAIST MEASUREMENT

▓▓ HIP MEASUREMENT

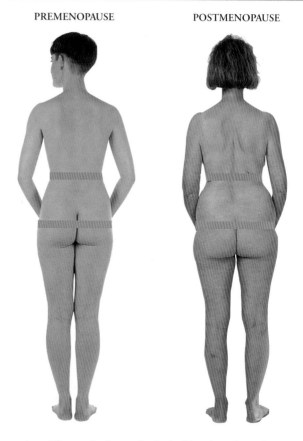

PREMENOPAUSE

POSTMENOPAUSE

running, if you don't particularly like the idea of exercise classes. If you already have heart problems, consult your doctor before starting an exercise regimen.

EMOTIONAL SYMPTOMS

Feelings such as tension, anxiety, depression, listlessness, irritability, and mood swings can occur at any age, but they rarely occur together or as frequently as they do during menopause. This is because the centers in the brain that control your sense of well-being, a positive state of mind, and a feeling of control and tranquility are all affected by the absence of estrogen, so for many women, menopausal mood changes resemble a roller coaster ride. Women describe subtle sensations such as trembling, fluttering, unease, and discomfort. More severe feelings of anxiety or panic can arise with little or no provocation. Tasks that you used to be able to tackle easily can now leave you in total panic. Mood swings from wild elation to deep despondency are quite common, and patience can be all too easily exhausted. The future may look bleak, your loss of self-esteem is precipitous, and you may feel truly depressed.

Depression, although rare, can strike during your menopausal years. This is distinct from any other emotional symptoms that you may experience such as tearfulness and anxiety. The following are all possible predictors of depression:

- Past or recent history of stressful events.
- Surgically induced menopause.
- Negative expectations of menopause.
- Severe hot flashes and night sweats.
- Family history of depressive illness.

Depression can be a debilitating illness that can last for weeks, months, or even years if left untreated. As a woman, you're more likely to experience depression than a man. Consult your doctor for professional help if you have experienced four of these symptoms for at least two weeks:

- Extreme eating patterns, such as bingeing.
- Unusual sleeping patterns.
- Being exceptionally lethargic or restless.
- An inability to enjoy a once pleasurable activity, including loss of sex drive.
- Debilitating fatigue or loss of energy.
- Feelings of worthlessness and self-reproach.
- Difficulty in concentrating and making even simple decisions.
- Thoughts of death or suicide, or suicide attempts (seek help right away).

COMPLEMENTARY THERAPY

Herbs that may have a calming effect are passion flower and valerian root. Passion flower helps insomnia and elevates the levels of serotonin in the blood, which creates a feeling of well-being. Adding an infusion of your favorite herbs to bathwater can also be therapeutic.

Menopausal depression may be alleviated by ginger root, cayenne pepper, dandelion root, and Siberian ginseng, all of which may work because they contain essential nutrients. Ginseng can have a tonic effect, and Siberian ginseng and liquorice root are also considered to be very effective in combating lassitude and depression.

EMOTIONAL SELF-HELP

Emotional symptoms will be easier to control if you follow the guidelines below.

- *Share your feelings with your partner. Severe mood swings and irritability can distance you from your partner and can jeopardize a relationship.*

- *Think about joining a self-help group or starting one yourself. Women who go to these groups may be better able to deal with depression.*

NATURAL PROGESTERONE

In the last few years there has been much media hype about the effectiveness of so-called "natural" progesterone for the treatment of menopausal symptoms. Lost in the hype, several important scientific facts have been ignored.

• *It is not natural to give progesterone for menopausal symptoms nor is it scientifically or medically logical. Menopause symptoms are related to lack of estrogen; progesterone in whatever form will not affect them.*

• *The original research work on progesterone for menopause certainly does not show that it is useful for menopausal women.*

• *Advocates of natural progesterone claim it is beneficial for osteoporosis (see p. 28), but the National Osteoporosis Foundation (NOF) opposes this view.*

• *It is claimed we are bombarded by xeno-estrogens in packaging, plastics, foods, and pesticides so we need progesterone to restore the balance – an idea that is at best no more than conjecture.*

DIET AND EXERCISE

Exercise can help hot flashes and night sweats, which can often be a contributing factor to menopausal emotional problems and depression. A good workout can lift your mood and produce an "exercise high" that can last up to eight hours. Try to have 20–30 minutes of short and sustained bouts of vigorous activity every morning to help you through the day. Relaxation techniques and meditation can promote tranquility and combat anxiety and tension. They can also improve suppleness and are worth trying on a regular basis (see tips on p. 42). Yoga, with its unique combination of exercise and relaxation techniques, could also work well (see p. 80).

INTELLECTUAL SYMPTOMS

Forgetfulness is one of the most common symptoms that menopausal women complain of, and they may experience it long before they stop menstruating. You may forget where you put something, you may miss appointments, and things that used to be simple to remember can suddenly require enormous effort. The ability to concentrate can also become difficult. These problems combined often make it hard to carry out work that involves complex assessments and major decision-making. Even minor decisions can sometimes be paralyzing.

DIET AND EXERCISE

Relatively little research has been conducted on the effect that nutrients have on intellectual processes, but there is some evidence that vitamins such as B_1 and B_{12} and minerals like calcium and potassium may all contribute to brain health. All of these are easy to incorporate into a normal healthy diet (see p. 50 and p. 52 for lists of vitamin- and mineral-rich foods). Bear in mind, however, that most vitamins need to be taken in conjunction with other vitamins and minerals in order to be absorbed by the body. A shortage of one vital element can cause the others to be less effective (see pp. 48–55 for further information).

Regular exercise also helps you feel more alert and less sluggish, and can improve concentration too. A brisk walk in the fresh air every day for at least 20 minutes will get you in shape mentally as well as physically.

2

MENOPAUSAL MEDICAL COMPLAINTS

As a result of the falling levels of estrogen during
menopause, combined with the natural aging
process in the postmenopausal years,
women can become increasingly susceptible
to illness. One of the most painful conditions
is osteoporosis, but there are also other serious
conditions, all of which can be overcome or
controlled with a combination of medical
and self-help measures.

OSTEOPOROSIS

A painful, crippling, and life-threatening condition, osteoporosis is the single most important health hazard for women past menopause – it is more common than heart disease, stroke, diabetes, or breast cancer. In its early stages, it has no obvious symptoms, so many women may be unaware that they have it. Because of the life-threatening nature of osteoporosis, it is vital that every woman be told the facts about this disease; women must become vigilant and take measures to prevent osteoporosis from destroying their lives.

The clinical definition of osteoporosis is "a condition where there is less normal bone than expected for a woman's age, with an increased risk of fracture." However, some experts use the term "osteoporosis" to describe low bone density where fractures have already occurred.

WHY IT HAPPENS

As estrogen and progesterone levels fall, bones begin to lose mass by 0.5–3 percent a year. By the time a woman is 80, she can easily have lost 40 percent of the bone mass in her body.

Estrogen facilitates the uptake of calcium from the blood into the bone and inhibits its loss. A fall in estrogen levels, therefore, leads to bone disintegration.

For a woman with severe osteoporosis of the spine, even minor blows, jolts, or falls can cause the spinal bones to fracture.

BONE DENSITY TESTS

There are several different ways of assessing bone density, and a scan is considered the best predictor of fracture. Bone density tests measure the density of the spine, wrist, and other high-risk areas. A decrease in bone mineral density (BMD) measured in the spine or the hip may indicate a 200 percent increase in the chance of any fracture, and a staggering 300 percent increase in the chance of a hip fracture.

PHYSICAL THERAPY

Physical therapy is often overlooked, but it should be an important part of your treatment for osteoporosis. A home exercise program can be established to continue the treatment. Increased muscle strength, improved spinal power and posture, maintenance of bone strength, relief of pain, and toning of pelvic floor muscles to cope with stress incontinence are all benefits of physical therapy.

Physical therapists may also use various forms of electrotherapy or ultrasound to help relieve pain. Some now also use complementary techniques such as acupuncture, and recommend the use of heating pads, hot-water bottles, or ice packs at home. TENS (Transcutaneous Electrical Nerve Stimulation) machines are available in most treatment centers for pain relief.

PREVENTING OSTEOPOROSIS

Since we are all at risk of developing osteoporosis, it is important that we adopt self-help measures to build up our natural resistance. Fortunately, there are a number of ways in which we can change our lifestyles to help maintain healthy bones.

Regular exercise, a balanced diet, and mental alertness can help to maintain overall fitness, and you should also have regular health checkups with your doctor.

Where possible, reduce the hazards in your home by removing any electrical cords and loose rugs that can cause you to trip. Make sure that there is always a firm banister on stairs and be particularly careful when walking on slippery or uneven surfaces.

Women who exercise twice a week have denser bones than those who only exercise once a week, who, in turn, have denser bones than those who never exercise at all. It is never too late to improve your body. Bones can be strengthened to resist the effect of estrogen depletion during the postmenopausal years.

Eat a calcium-rich diet The most important dietary advice for the early prevention of osteoporosis is to eat calcium-rich foods (see p. 52 for examples of calcium-rich foods). In brief, to prevent your bones from becoming brittle, you need calcium for bone mass, vitamin D to absorb the calcium into your body, and estrogen to maintain the calcium inside your bones.

Common fracture sites
Women with osteoporosis characteristically suffer from fractures of the wrists, hip bones, vertebrae, pelvis, and shoulder bones.

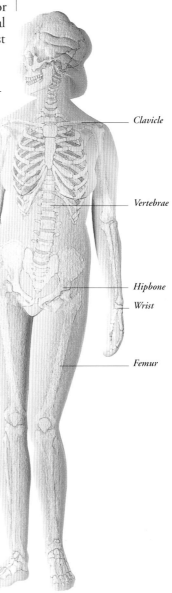

Clavicle

Vertebrae

Hipbone

Wrist

Femur

HEART ATTACKS AND STROKES

Heart attacks and strokes stem from a disease of the arteries that narrows the artery channels, reduces blood flow, and increases blood pressure (see below). Arteries become coated by fat and prone to blockage.

RISK FACTORS

Your chances of suffering from disease of the arteries are increased by obesity, smoking, lack of exercise, high blood pressure, and being menopausal and postmenopausal. Women who develop heart disease after menopause should pay particular attention to the risk factors under their control, such as smoking, diet, and stress levels.

When blood flow becomes impeded – generally after a number of years – you may experience angina, which is pain in the chest on exertion, or intermittent claudi-cation, which is leg pain brought on by walking and alleviated by rest. If blood flow is restricted in the arteries supplying the brain, you may experience temporary stroke symptoms, dizziness, and fainting attacks. Kidney failure is also possible if the renal artery becomes narrowed.

PREVENTION

Lowering risk factors, especially in early adulthood and midlife, can help prevent disease of the arteries from developing. You should try to give up smoking, have your blood pressure checked regularly, and get high blood pressure treated. Keep your diet low in saturated fats, and if your cholesterol levels still remain high, you may need medication. Regular exercise is essential.

HIGH BLOOD PRESSURE

Measurements for blood pressure are expressed as two figures: for example, 120/80. A blood pressure that is consistently above 160/95 is considered high.

An increase in blood pressure occurs when there is resistance in the blood vessels to the flow of blood. Resistance rises in the large blood vessels because of increased rigidity due to age, and occurs in the small blood vessels when they become constricted in response to nerve impulses or hormones.

RISK FACTORS

Apart from being postmenopausal, other risk factors for essential hypertension (high blood pressure) include smoking, obesity, excessive alcohol consumption, a family history of high blood pressure, a sedentary life-style, stress, and old age.

SELF-HELP

High blood pressure can often be reduced by making changes in your life style. If you smoke, you should quit or at the very least cut down (see p. 64). You should also assess your alcohol intake. If you are a heavy drinker you should cut down drastically or try to stop drinking altogether (see pp. 64–65). If you are overweight, you should try to lose weight (see p. 56) and exercise more (see pp. 58–63). Dietary measures could include cutting down on salt intake and eating less fatty food (see Good Nutrition, pp. 48–55).

Biofeedback training can be helpful to some patients in reducing their blood pressure. This involves learning a variety of breathing and relaxation techniques. During a biofeedback session your blood pressure is continuously monitored and you learn to respond immediately to any increase in blood pressure by practicing breathing and relaxation techniques.

STROKE

This is a potentially fatal result of hypertension (high blood pressure). Sixty percent of strokes are caused by a cerebral thrombosis, when an artery in the brain becomes blocked by a clot (thrombus) that has built up in its wall.

About a third of major strokes are fatal. A third result in some disability with speech or movement and a third have no long-term ill effects. Strokes are rare before the age of 60, but thereafter the risk increases rapidly.

SELF-HELP

After hospital treatment, stroke patients spend most of their recovery period at home relearning how to use the parts of their body that may have been paralyzed. There are many self-help aids available that can make life easier, such as easy-to-hold utensils. Dressing in front of a mirror may speed up relearning.

The classic symptoms of cystitis are listed below.

• *The frequent, urgent need to urinate.*

• *Severe pain when you do urinate.*

• *A dragging pain in the lower abdomen.*

• *Very rarely, the presence of blood in the urine.*

UROGENITAL AGING

When estrogen is plentiful, the bladder, urethra, and vagina stay healthy. When hormone levels fall during menopause the urogenital system thins, atrophies, and becomes susceptible to infection.

SYMPTOMS

Signs of genital atrophy include a dry, itchy vagina and vulva, which causes pain during sex. These symptoms are often combined with the frequent, urgent desire to urinate, and incontinence. This combination of symptoms, known as urogenital syndrome, is the most common reason for women over the age of 55 to visit a gynecologist.

CYSTITIS

Estrogen is so crucial to the health of the urinary tract that after menopause the bladder is far more vulnerable to bacterial infection. Cystitis, inflammation of the inner lining of the bladder, is most commonly caused by *Escherichia coli* (*E. coli*) bacterium.

SELF-HELP

Drink lots of water or diluted fruit juice at the beginning of an attack. *E. coli* cannot multiply in alkaline urine, and you can make your urine alkaline by taking a teaspoon of baking soda in a glass of water. Drink this three times within five hours of the first twinge of pain. Soluble aspirin and a hot-water bottle can provide some relief.

Each time you urinate, wash your hands afterward. You should also wipe your perineum from front to back once with a damp cotton ball. Soap and water can dry out the perineum and vagina and make you more prone to infection. When you dry yourself, pat gently.

If your cystitis is provoked by intercourse, it is probably best to refrain from sex until you are more comfortable. Otherwise, reduce friction with a lubricating jelly and experiment to find the most comfortable sexual position. You should also wash carefully and urinate after sex.

PRURITIS VULVAE

Itching is a sign of estrogen deficiency, and pruritis vulvae – chronic, uncontrollable itching of the vaginal area – is usually worst in hot weather or during the night. Diabetes, vaginal yeast infections such as thrush, and urinary tract infections can all cause pruritis vulvae. However, it can be pyschogenic in origin. Repeated scratching can become more and more pleasurable, even to the point of orgasm. Eventually the sufferer will develop profound soreness and thickening of the skin in the vaginal area.

SELF-HELP

You can prevent pruritis vulvae from getting worse by trying not to scratch the vaginal area. Consult your doctor if it persists for more than two days – if you don't, you may find yourself in an unbreakable itch-scratch-itch cycle. Pay particular attention to normal hygiene but, if possible, avoid the use of soap and detergents, which will strip the skin of oils and make it more sensitive. Use only warm or cool water, and try applying a silicone-based hand cream to the itchy area after each washing. Ice packs may also help to numb the itch. Don't use local anesthetic creams and sprays because these may cause allergic reactions.

INCONTINENCE

This occurs when the sphincter muscle at the base of your bladder becomes so weak (or the bladder muscle becomes overactive) that you have little or no control over the flow of urine. There are several different types of incontinence – see right for the most common.

SELF-HELP

Mild incontinence is often due to weakened pelvic floor muscles, and you can improve your bladder control by doing Kegel exercises. These involve repeatedly contracting and relaxing the muscles of the urogenital tract (see p. 14). If you are suffering from urge incontinence, self-help measures include emptying your bladder every two hours, and avoiding diuretic drinks, such as tea and coffee. There are a number of aids available for incontinence sufferers. These include waterproof bedsheets, incontinence pads, female urinals, and waterproof pants. However, you should consult your doctor long before these become necessary. If you suffer from stress incontinence when you exercise, try emptying your bladder beforehand. Wearing a tampon during exercise can act as a splint to the urethra.

TYPES OF INCONTINENCE

The following are the three most common types of incontinence.

Stress incontinence *This is the leakage of a small amount of urine caused by an increase in pressure inside the abdomen when you sneeze, cough, laugh, or lift a heavy object.*

Urge incontinence *This occurs if you wait until you need to urinate urgently. The bladder starts to contract involuntarily and empties itself. This type of incontinence is often triggered by a sudden change in position, such as standing up.*

Mixed pattern incontinence *This is a combination of both urge and stress incontinence, and may be the result of two faults in the bladder function.*

MEDIUM TO HIGH RISK FACTORS

The following conditions can make you more prone to breast cancer.

- *Having a family history of breast cancer (especially close female relatives).*
- *Early onset of menstruation and late menopause.*
- *Being over the age of 40.*
- *Having children later than average.*
- *Being Caucasian.*
- *Obesity or a diet high in animal or dairy fat.*

LOW RISK FACTORS

The following conditions will make you less prone to breast cancer.

- *Having several children.*
- *Breast-feeding.*
- *Being short and thin.*
- *Late onset of menstruation and early menopause.*

BREAST CANCER

This is the most common type of cancer in women, and is the leading cause of death in women aged between 35 and 55. In the US, women have a one in nine lifetime chance of developing breast cancer.

MEDICAL TREATMENT

Most doctors will refer a woman with a breast lump to a hospital so that further tests can be done. If you have a cyst, the fluid can be removed and examined, and a clear-cut diagnosis made.

If the lump is small and shallow it is possible to have an outpatient lumpectomy. The lump is removed with some surrounding tissue and then examined in the laboratory. If cancer is discovered, blood tests, X rays, and bone scans will be carried out to help decide upon the right treatment.

Radical treatments, such as mastectomy, do not necessarily improve survival rates. Many surgeons now recommend lumpectomy combined with radiation therapy or anticancer medicines (chemotherapy).

OUTLOOK

If a very small tumor is treated early, a complete cure is likely. All women who have had breast cancer will be asked to have regular checkups to detect any recurrence or spread of the cancer to the rest of the body. It is very important to perform regular breast self-examinations (see p. 21) and have annual mammograms starting at age 40. Even if the cancer recurs, it can be controlled for many years with surgery, medicines, and radiation.

TYPES OF COMMON BREAST SURGERY

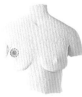

Lumpectomy
The whole lump and a small area of surrounding tissue is removed.

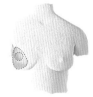

Partial Mastectomy
Removal of a substantial area of the breast tissue and the nipple.

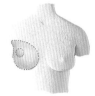

Extended Mastectomy
All of the breast is removed plus some lymph nodes from the armpit.

3

POSITIVE ATTITUDES

Menopause is sometimes incorrectly stereotyped as the start of a gradual decline into old age, when your body loses its feminine qualities and becomes sexually inactive. Women know from experience that this is far from the truth. With care, your body remains one to be proud of, your mental resilience continues to be great, and you still have a valuable role to play in society. By adopting a positive attitude to life in general, and to your changing lifestyle and body in particular, you can improve the quality of your life and be living proof that this is only the end of the beginning, not the beginning of the end.

Try to act on the following positive statements:

• *Being well-informed helps me to deal effectively with any menopausal symptoms that arise.*

• *The speed of aging does not accelerate after menopause.*

• *Femininity is not dependent on fertility.*

• *I deserve understanding from my partner and family.*

• *If I experience menopausal symptoms, I talk about them. The more open I am, the more I will help to break down taboos.*

• *I have the right to take control of my life. If I don't want to rely on doctors or medicine, I won't. There are good relaxation techniques as well as complementary and dietary approaches that can help deal successfully with any symptoms.*

• *I can take steps to maintain and even improve the quality of my sex life (see p. 81). There is no reason why menopause should be the beginning of a sexual decline.*

• *There's no time like the present for developing a new skill, hobby, or project. I can even begin a second career.*

• *I will start financial planning for retirement as early as possible, to take advantage of what could be my most creative years.*

THINKING POSITIVELY

Referring to menopause as the change of life can be misleading and counterproductive. Menopause isn't the only change that will occur during your life and it is unlikely to be the most significant one. Life is a whole series of gradual changes – we don't suddenly reach a turning point and start growing old when we reach midlife. Aging is a continuous process that begins the moment we are born and continues until we die. I believe a healthy attitude about menopause is to see it as a time in which to rediscover yourself, to assess (or reassess) your life and its purpose, and to establish new goals.

By the time we reach middle age, most of us carry around the received wisdom of society, leftovers from old traditions, fears that can be obsolete, and beliefs that may be borrowed. Without clearing out all these redundant feelings, we can lose touch with our inner selves.

RESISTING NEGATIVE STEREOTYPES

It is important to resist negative stereotypes associated with menopause. These are very often culturally created and do not reflect the reality of our individual experiences. In countries where age is venerated and older women are respected for their experience and wisdom, fewer physical and psychological symptoms of menopause are reported. In countries that lack a tradition of myths and misconceptions about menopause, aging seems to be regarded as a more natural process; women aren't adversely affected by negative images and may feel less confused by what is happening to them.

If you believe that in order to be beautiful and successful you must be young, then you may not enjoy your middle age to the fullest. If you are convinced that the quality of life deteriorates from the age of 50 onward, this can become a self-fulfilling prophecy. Since you believe it is going to happen, you may inadvertently make it happen by not taking care of yourself and by adopting resigned, negative attitudes.

TAKING CONTROL OF YOUR BODY

The first step toward taking charge of your life and managing menopause is to take charge of your body. You need to play an active role with all of your medical and health providers. Be aware of all your options and exercise them in order to eliminate as many health problems as you can. The strategy you choose to deal with any menopausal symptoms you may suffer from is up to you. You could decide to try self-help measures, for instance, or complementary medicine. Alternatively, you may feel that your symptoms warrant conventional medical help.

To achieve these goals, you need to have a firm sense of your own self-worth and optimism about the future, and you must be prepared to make an effort. As soon as you start to take control of your menopausal symptoms, your health and sense of well-being will benefit enormously.

TAKING CONTROL OF YOUR MIND

The second step toward taking charge of your life and managing your menopause is to take charge of your mind. As with your body, you need to be positive in your attitude and prepared to make a real effort to get what you want from both your family and friends, and from medical and other professionals with whom you come into contact. Try to keep in mind the positive statements listed on the left – and remember that menopause is not the beginning of the end; it's the beginning of the rest of your life.

THE POWER OF POSITIVE THINKING

While health and vigor during the menopausal years depend a great deal on following a good diet and doing plenty of exercise, these are by no means the only resources you have to draw upon. Rest, relaxation, and a variety of leisure activities will help you keep active and mentally alert. You also need self-affirming thoughts to maintain your self-confidence and prevent self-criticism. Never allow yourself to think that you are unattractive, lackluster, or out-of-touch. The strong interaction between your mind and your body allows you to make menopause more difficult with negative thoughts. In other words, if you believe you're sick, you can start to behave like a sick person.

If you try to repeat some of the statements on the right like a mantra each day, you will gradually become more and more convinced of their truth.

A PERSONAL MANTRA

Positive thoughts and attitudes will maintain your self-esteem.

- *My body is strong and healthy and can become healthier each day.*

- *My female organs are in good shape.*

- *My body chemistry is effective and balanced.*

- *I eat healthy, nourishing food.*

- *I'm learning to handle stress.*

- *I'm calm and relaxed.*

- *I work efficiently and competently.*

- *I have the freedom and confidence to enjoy life.*

- *I can be happy and optimistic at this time of my life.*

- *My life belongs to me and it brings me pleasure.*

- *I devote time to myself each day.*

- *My friends and family are more enjoyable than they have ever been.*

- *I'm going through menopause more easily and more comfortably with each passing day.*

CHANGING FAMILY ROLES

The structure of the family is constantly changing. For many of us, the time when we really need stability and continuity may be the very time when we may have to cope with a major upheaval in the family, such as a divorce, remarriage, and new relations with various children and children-in-law. As we get older, we may have to decide with whom or near whom we are going to live.

The extended families that can arise from divorce and remarriage may include young adults who have grown up with the idea that their parents are fixed points in the universe. Suddenly they may acquire new grandparents. Similarly, grandparents may find themselves with new grandchildren. At first, this may be hard to deal with, but people often overcome these difficulties through love and generosity. Newly formed family ties can be just as strong as old ones.

CARING FOR ELDERLY PARENTS

Although family relationships have changed radically in the last century, one thing that has remained fairly consistent is the way in which younger members of a family assume responsibility for older ones. There is no doubt that this can place severe emotional, physical, and economic stress on us. The mobility of today's society means that the family is not always gathered in one place. Even a few minutes' traveling time can make support difficult, especially if we have other commitments, such as work.

Sometimes the responsibilities of looking after home, husband, and aged parents, as well as dealing with postmenopausal symptoms, can be overwhelming. Try to delegate as much as you can. Enlist the help of your partner, children, and siblings. If you have a very old, infirm parent, you may have to decide to house him or her in a nursing home or other facility. No family should feel guilty about this – it's a responsible option, making sure that your parent is well cared for.

BECOMING A GRANDPARENT

One of the joys that many people have in store for them in midlife is becoming a grandparent. Once past childbearing age, many women begin to look forward to their second chance at mothering and find that few experiences compare with spending time, learning from, and teaching their grandchildren. In my opinion, grandparents are an important part of the family; they can teach a child how to relate to older people. Grandparents, by virtue of their age, may be more philosophical, tolerant, and sympathetic than parents. Over many years of practice they have learned the knack of handling children with ease. These qualities enable children to develop in a relaxed, familiar environment.

It's sometimes said that grandparents spoil their grandchildren. This must be a misuse of the word "spoil." If spoiling a child means giving him explanations instead of dismissals, suggesting alternatives instead of negatives, and helping him instead of ignoring him, then grandparents do indeed spoil children. As a grandparent you are in a position to share your passions with your grandchildren, whether they be gardening, sewing, sketching, or swimming. As grandchildren grow up, you can be a valuable confidante to them. You, of all people, are best equipped to teach them how they can cope with change, having lived through some of the most dramatic upheavals the world has known. You have a valuable historical perspective on employment, politics, and social change. Recount your past experiences and encourage them to ask you questions.

You can provide a positive role model of middle and old age for your family. You can be independent. You can also listen. Parents don't always have a lot of time for this, but you are in a position to listen to family members without giving advice. You can tell your family about your own experience and what it has led you to believe.

You may find that you have much more in common with teenage grandchildren than you had ever imagined. At opposite ends of life, you are likely to be experiencing changing identities and asking the same questions: Who am I? What do I really want? How do I get it? Very frequently adolescents can have more in common with grandparents than with parents, who are too busy to be self-aware and introspective. Grandparents can give a unique kind of loving and caring, and grandchildren relish knowing that they hold a special place in their grandparents' lives.

ROLE OF GRANDMOTHERS

You can maximize your enjoyment of your grandchildren by acting on the following advice.

- *Find free time to talk and listen to your grandchildren.*

- *Find time to spend on activities that are fun, rather than routine.*

- *Live apart from grandchildren, allowing the children to feel they have a second home.*

- *Provide personal information to daughters or daughters-in-law from your own experience.*

- *Have an overview about general child care.*

- *Create more time for mothers by taking care of children.*

MENTAL AGILITY

Most of us are concerned about our physical fitness, but fewer of us stop to consider our mental fitness. Women, regardless of their marital status, suffer more from mental illness than men and can become even more vulnerable around the time of menopause. During middle age, some women feel that their freedom of choice becomes more restricted, and this can lead to frustration, conflict, unhappiness, and mental trauma.

Mental fitness can be as easy to develop as physical fitness. We must strive to maintain a basic level of mental health so that we can rise to cope with any challenges that present themselves, deal with emergencies, and generally have the resilience to survive stressful situations in the long-term. As we get older, we have to deal with emotional trauma, such as the loss of parents and possibly our partner.

Self-knowledge requires supreme realism: we have to learn that we are not unique in suffering, that difficult times come and go, that adversity is normal, and that some failures are inevitable. As we grow older, we should leave behind preconceptions and prejudices, and be constantly prepared to change our attitudes. We need to work with our emotions in a constructive way, and yet still be affectionate and tender with ourselves.

STAYING MENTALLY FIT

We can learn a lot by observing the qualities of people whose mental and emotional resiliency we admire. The following qualities come from emotional openness, flexibility, and self-reliance.

• Independence and recognition of others' independence, privacy, and peace.

• Lack of self-pity, so that when a problem arises it is looked at objectively.

• The attitude that nothing is hopeless and problems are there to be solved.

• A sense of inner security rather than security gained from controlling others.

• Being prepared to take responsibility for our own mistakes.

• A few close and loving relationships rather than many superficial ones.

- A sense of realism about the goals we set ourselves.
- Being in touch with our emotions and feeling free to express them.

Just as a muscle becomes weak if it's not exercised regularly, so your brain will slow and become feeble if it is not stimulated. The best mental exercise is work. A recent experiment performed on Japanese octogenarians showed that those who kept going into their offices, even for one hour a day, had greater mental powers than those who had retired at 60 and given up disciplined thinking.

The first tip to maintain mental fitness is daily intellectual work. It helps if your efforts are judged by your peers, but work of any kind provides mental stimulation. Interaction with other people forces you to assess what they are saying and respond with questions and comments. Your brain has to assimilate information and your cognitive processes remain active.

As we get older, we lose the ability to form new brain connections, so we have to make certain that old and well-established connections are continually used. The only way to do this is through thinking. Don't make the mistake of believing that thinking is a passive process – it means engaging in, questioning, and absorbing what is happening all around us. For example, arithmetical "exercises" are often encountered in daily life and you can engage in them more actively. Anticipate your supermarket bill by adding up the cost of your shopping or estimate how much change you'll receive. Try to judge the size and quantity of objects and then measure them to check on your judgment.

Try to add to your vocabulary daily by noting down each new word you see or hear. Keep a dictionary handy to check on meanings and use the word in subsequent conversations. Read a daily newspaper article or watch the news on television and discuss the main events of the day with a friend.

If you have the opportunity, think about taking an evening class. The range of courses available to adults is huge – there are crafts courses that take up a couple of hours a week, or you can take full-time courses in academic subjects such as history or American literature. Your local library is the best source of information on continuing education.

MEMORY MAINTENANCE

Follow the simple measures below to improve your memory.

- *When you read a book or magazine article, summarize the plot or the points made in it to a friend.*

- *When you're going shopping, try to collect as many items as possible without referring to your shopping list.*

- *If you want to remember several things, do it with a mnemonic. For example, you can abbreviate tasks such as ironing, making a phone call, and typing a letter into the single word PIT (Phone/Iron/Type), which will act as a memory aid.*

- *If you walk into a room and forget why you're there, go back to where you came from and don't leave until you have remembered.*

- *If you have lost something, track it down. Write down the last six things you did prior to losing it and where you were for each activity. Draw a grid with what you were doing along one side and where you were along the bottom. The item you've lost lies in one of those squares; check each one out until you find it.*

DEEP-MUSCLE RELAXATION

Follow the steps below to relax your body.

1 Find a peaceful place, lie on your back, or sit in a comfortable chair and close your eyes.

2 Tense your right hand (or left, if you are left-handed), then let it go loose. Imagine it feels heavy and warm. Repeat with your right forearm, upper arm, and shoulder, then move onto the right foot, lower leg, upper leg. Now do exactly the same thing with the left side of your body. By the time you have finished, your hands, arms, and legs should feel heavy, relaxed, and warm. Allow a few seconds for these feelings to develop and to get used to the sensation.

3 Now relax the muscles around your hips and waist. Let the relaxation flow up the abdomen into the chest. You will find that your breathing starts to slow down.

4 Let the relaxation go into your shoulders, facial, and jaw muscles. Pay special attention to the muscles around your eyes and forehead – tense them, then let the frown melt away. Finish by imagining that your forehead feels cool and smooth.

RELAXATION

If you are relaxed, you will be better able to deal with problems and conflicts at home and work, and you will find personal relationships easier to manage. Irritability and aggressiveness will dissipate and you will find you have energy to spare. Relaxation can often help you deal with menopausal symptoms such as hot flashes.

DEEP-MUSCLE RELAXATION

The deep-muscle technique described on the left has been used by most relaxation experts around the world. It may take time to learn, but it will help you cope with stress, lower your blood pressure, decrease your chances of getting headaches, and make you sleep better.

If you can, practice this technique twice a day for 15–20 minutes each time. However, even as little as three minutes will be sufficient time to give you a sense of well-being. The best time to practice is just before mealtimes or an hour afterward.

DEEP-MENTAL RELAXATION

Once you've mastered deep-muscle relaxation, you're ready to go on to deep-mental relaxation (see opposite). This technique is designed to clear your mind of stressful thoughts and tension. It is a form of meditation in which you attempt to separate your body from your thoughts in order to create a personal space that is free from worry and negative thoughts. You can retreat or escape to this whenever you want to. Find a place where you know you will not be disturbed and lie down or make yourself comfortable in a chair. Before you start the steps themselves, close your eyes and begin by breathing deeply several times.

When you've mastered both deep-muscle and deep-mental relaxation, they can be done together. They're fairly easy to combine, and you should practice them twice a day until you become competent.

INSTANT RELAXATION

Once you have trained your body to achieve deep-muscle and mental relaxation, you should be able to achieve partial relaxation within about 30 seconds. If you are feeling stressed, try the following exercise.

Sit, lie, or stand comfortably. Take a deep breath to the count of five, then breathe out slowly and tell your muscles to relax. Repeat three times until you're feeling relaxed. Imagine yourself in a pleasant situation, such as walking along a beach. If a situation panics you, regain control by breathing deeply. This should calm you and lessen the stress.

MENTAL IMAGERY

Use your imagination to get in touch with your body. For example, focus on your left hand and make it feel warm. Now concentrate on your right thigh and make it feel warm and heavy. Try to imagine that one leg is heavier than the other. Once you've mastered this, you can apply it in any situation by imagining that your body has the inner resources to overcome the symptoms you are experiencing. As part of cancer therapy, patients are trained to imagine their body's defenses as warriors, physically killing their cancer cells. You can use this technique to combat menopausal symptoms.

BREATHING TECHNIQUES

Almost all muscle relaxation programs involve proper breathing as the key to controlling stress and anxiety. This may be simple deep breathing, yoga breathing, or deep abdominal breathing.

Most people breathe incorrectly, using no more than a third of their lung capacity, and hardly using the abdomen at all. Most of us only use the upper part of the chest, so we are depriving the body of oxygen. Try to change your shallow breathing to deep, slow breathing. Besides improving the function of your lungs and the muscles of your abdomen, it will relax your whole body.

To do deep abdominal breathing, place one hand on your stomach and breathe in slowly through your nose to a count of five. As you inhale, let it balloon out. The farther out it goes, the more lung capacity you use, and the more oxygen you are getting to your tissues. When you think your lungs are absolutely full, try to take a little more air into the very bottom of your lungs. Then breathe out deeply, through your nose if you can, but through your mouth if it allows your stomach and chest to collapse completely. This "oxygen fix" is wonderfully refreshing and you can do it as often as you like.

DEEP-MENTAL RELAXATION

Follow the steps below to relax your mind.

1 Allow thoughts to associate freely in your head.

2 Stop any recurring thoughts by saying "no" to them under your breath, and repeating "no" until they go away.

3 With your eyes closed, imagine a tranquil scene such as a calm, blue sea. Whatever you imagine, try to see the color blue because this is very therapeutic.

4 Concentrate on your breathing – and make sure it is slow and natural. Follow each breath as you inhale and exhale.

5 By now, you should feel calm and rested. You may find it helpful to repeat a soothing mantra such as "love," "peace," or "calm."

6 Remind yourself to keep the muscles of your face, eyes, and forehead relaxed, and imagine that your forehead is cool and smooth.

YOUR APPEARANCE

Many women first become really conscious of the signs of aging on their faces and bodies during menopause. It is very important to feel comfortable with the way you look – not only will your confidence improve but your whole outlook will also benefit. A feeling of self-esteem is particularly important as you get older, and looking after your appearance is a very good way of promoting self-worth.

Your body will look better if you eat a healthy diet containing the right vitamins and minerals (see pp. 48–52) and exercise regularly. You can make the most of your skin and hair if you take proper care of them. Paying attention to your figure will mean not only that your clothes fit more comfortably but that they will look more flattering too.

There's no secret formula for looking good. You have to think carefully and logically about how to make the most of your good points and how to conceal your bad ones successfully. There's absolutely no need to buy expensive cosmetics or clothes; it's much more important to look natural and feel comfortable. The truly wonderful thing about reaching menopause is that there are no prescribed roles for you to play, and no set rules that you have to follow.

POSTURE

Shapelessness and poor posture can give the impression of age, and a relaxed, upright posture and a supple figure can make you look much younger. Bad posture can also make you look fat (or at least fatter), while good posture can take pounds off as well as years. Make sure that you stand with your feet parallel, your pelvis straight, and your spine vertical. Your shoulders should be relaxed rather than hunched. You will not only improve your appearance by paying attention to your posture and gait, but you will help maintain the health of your spine, and back muscles.

CLOTHES

If you remain in good shape, there's nothing to prevent you from continuing to wear the kind of clothes you have always worn. However, aging inevitably brings changes to body shape, and you may want to accommodate these. Comfortable good-quality garments with flattering lines suit mature women, but you should avoid viewing your age as a constraint upon what you should and shouldn't wear.

If you suffer from hot flashes or night sweats, avoid synthetic fabrics such as polyester or nylon and wear cooling, natural ones such as cotton. It may also be wiser to avoid wearing wool next to your skin, although it is a natural fabric. And don't wear tightly fitting garments whatever the material – they'll make you sweat even more.

Choose your shoes very carefully too. High heels can throw your body out of alignment and increase the likelihood of falling. Shoes that are too narrow will cramp your toes and cause corns and ingrown toenails. When you are at home, make a point of taking your shoes and panty hose off and allowing your feet to spread and relax.

UNDERWEAR

Even if your waistline and hips start to spread, you shouldn't be tempted to wear rigid corsets. If you feel you must wear foundation garments, then choose light ones that allow you to move and breathe freely. Lightweight undergarments make hot flashes easier to cope with. If possible, wear underwear that is made of natural fibers such as cotton and silk, since these are the most comfortable fabrics to have next to your skin, particularly in hot weather. Avoid wearing harsh, coarse fabrics next to the skin, and look for fastenings that are easy to reach and operate.

Your underwear should always be chosen on the basis of comfort and fit. Make sure you choose a bra with wide straps that don't cut into your skin, and try wearing an underwired bra for extra support, particularly if you have large breasts. Two tips to remember when you are buying a bra: if it rides up and sits high on your back, this means that it is too big; if you cannot comfortably slide a finger underneath the straps at the front, then it is too small. You should also check carefully that there are no bulges of flesh around your cleavage; this is a good indication that the cup size is too small.

CHOOSING A BRA

Underwired bras give support and can prevent the appearance of sagging breasts. Make sure the wired part lies flat against your skin and extends underneath your arms. Choose a bra with wide, soft straps and no lace – lace digs into the skin and makes it sore.

HAIR SELF-HELP

Follow the steps below to perfect hair.

• *Do not scrub your scalp when you wash your hair. You will loosen hairs from the soft, wet hair follicles.*

• *Do not tug or pull at wet hair as you comb it; this will remove or tear it. Use a wide-toothed brush or comb.*

• *Do not brush or comb your hair too frequently, which may make it look lank and dull.*

• *Do not use antidandruff shampoos more than once every two weeks, because they contain ingredients that can irritate the scalp.*

YOUR HAIR

As you get older, new hair grows in with no pigment. Gray hair is just as healthy as pigmented hair and needs no special treatment. As far as general hair care is concerned, use the mildest shampoo you can find and shampoo your hair only once – shampoos are now so efficient that shampooing twice is unnecessary. Mix two teaspoonfuls of shampoo in a glass of warm water and pour it over your already wet hair. Then massage the shampoo very gently into your hair. It's not necessary to scrub hard to work up a lather, just leave the shampoo on for about a minute, and then rinse until the hair is clean. If your hair is slightly dry, you will need a conditioner; these work by coating, or softening and swelling, the hair fiber. After you have washed your hair, dab it dry with a towel rather than rubbing it vigorously.

Gray hair can be hidden with temporary or permanent coloring but, to avoid a harsh contrast with your skin, it's probably better to use a shade that is lighter than the original color of your hair. The way your hair responds to artificial colorants depends on how porous your hair shafts are. There are several types of coloring.

• Restorers can be combed through or sprayed on. They work by coating the hair, and eventually may make it brittle and easily damaged.

• Temporary color, dry or liquid, gives highlights to gray hair, but it doesn't last beyond one shampoo.

• Semipermanent color blends gray hairs into your natural color and completely covers them. It fades over a period of time, especially in the sun, so reapplication is necessary every few weeks.

• Permanent hair color penetrates the hair shaft itself and cannot be shampooed away. It has a chemical base that can dry out the hair. It also leaves a regrowth when new hair grows in, and has to be reapplied every four to six weeks depending on the rate of growth. Try to avoid bleach, since this strips the hair of natural oils.

Make sure your hair is regularly looked after, and pay as much as you can afford for a style that really suits you. Don't let yourself be pressured into expensive perms and colors. Gray hair can be very attractive and you may not want to go to the trouble of regular coloring.

PHYSICAL HEALTH

Monitoring and maintaining your health is the key to continuing a healthy, happy, and active life. Observing and reading the messages your body sends, and responding sensitively to them, bring a real sense of achievement as well as well-being. And there is simply no doubt about it: it is not difficult to enjoy natural good health. Eating healthy food *does* make you feel better; controlling your weight *does* make you look better; and keeping fit *does* make you more energetic. What's more, any efforts you make quickly become apparent, giving you the incentive to continue the good work.

GOOD NUTRITION

As you get older, your digestive tract becomes less efficient and digestion can take longer. Your body no longer finds it as easy to cope with foods that contain a lot of calories but little nourishment. Although you need fewer calories than you did when you were younger, you still require the same amount of vitamins and minerals. The healthiest diet during menopause, therefore, is one that consists of unprocessed fresh foods such as whole grains, vegetables, fruits, fish, seafood, some oils, and the occasional egg. A range of healthy foods is now widely available, so it has never been easier to experiment. Concentrate on building up a regular diet composed of unprocessed, high-grade carbohydrates to which protein can be added as a "condiment."

As your body's metabolism and chemical reactions slow down, an adequate intake of vitamins and minerals is essential. Eating the right diet can have a powerful and beneficial effect on menopausal symptoms, making you independent of doctors and medicines.

Some protein is essential for health, but too much, especially in the form of fatty meats, can lead to deficient calcium absorption. If you've been a heavy meat-eater in the past, this could increase your risk of developing the bone disease, osteoporosis (see p. 28). Start to cut down on the amount of meat in your diet as soon as possible and try to replace it with foods such as fish, rice, beans, vegetables, and pasta.

A certain amount of fat is needed for functions that cannot be performed by any other nutrient. Essential fatty acids are necessary for the metabolism of calcium, for instance, and they cannot be manufactured by the body. The best forms of fat are those found in whole natural foods such as vegetable oils and fish oils. Fats to avoid are saturated fats; that is, fats that are solid at room temperature – these include butter and lard, and certain vegetable oils, such as coconut or palm oil, found in processed foods.

Fermented milk products, such as yogurt, can be particularly effective at encouraging calcium absorption. Even those who have problems digesting whole-milk products can usually tolerate fermented ones because they are partially predigested.

BASIC ESSENTIALS

Vitamins, minerals, fiber, and water are some of the basic essentials of any diet. Making sure your diet contains adequate amounts of all of them should be one of your most important priorities. In addition to the general information listed below, see also the charts on p. 50 and p. 52 for specific guidance on vitamin- and mineral-rich foods, and how they can help you become healthier.

VITAMIN A

This is necessary for the health and growth of the skin, eyes, and mucous membranes. A vitamin A deficiency can cause night blindness and an increased susceptibility to infections. The lack of vitamin A may also contribute to heavy menstrual bleeding and to skin conditions related to the aging process.

VITAMIN B COMPLEX

Several B vitamins are useful during menopause. Their effects include helping us to handle sugar, keeping the liver healthy, and stabilizing brain function. Low levels can lead to emotional distress, fatigue, and irritability. Folic acid (another B vitamin) may help to prevent precancerous changes in the cervix. If you're taking hormone replacement therapy (HRT), you may want to take a vitamin B_6 supplement because HRT can lead to a deficiency that may make you prone to depression.

VITAMIN C

This is often dubbed the "healing" vitamin; it helps mend wounds and burns, and it maintains collagen, which helps lubricate the skin (see p. 17). To a degree, it could be called an antiwrinkle vitamin. Since the need for collagen regeneration increases with age, we need greater amounts of vitamin C as we grow older. Vitamin C also helps the adrenal glands and the body's immune system fight infections and allergies.

VITAMIN D

Along with calcium and estrogen, vitamin D is essential to maintain bone mass and prevent the onset of osteoporosis (see p. 28) after menopause. Vitamin D promotes the absorption of calcium and phosphorus from the intestine. All menopausal women should include adequate quantities of this vitamin in their diet to maintain strong, straight bones in later life.

VITAMIN E

Vitamin E has been used with some success as an estrogen substitute. It is possible that vitamin E may relieve hot flashes and the psychological symptoms of

VITAMINS THAT WILL BENEFIT MENOPAUSAL COMPLAINTS

VITAMIN	SOURCE	COMPLAINT
Vitamin A (Retinol and carotene)	Carrots, spinach, turnips, apricots, liver, cantaloupe, sweet potatoes	Excessive menstrual bleeding, cervical abnormalities, fibrocystic breast disease, breast cancer, leukoplakia, and other skin conditions
Folic Acid (Vitamin B complex)	Green leafy vegetables, nuts, peas, beans, liver, and kidney	Cervical abnormalities and cancer, osteoporosis, diabetes
Vitamin B_3 (Niacin)	Meat and poultry, fish, legumes, whole wheat, bran	Hyperlipidemia (high concentration of blood fat), hypoglycemia (low blood sugar)
Vitamin B_6 (Pyriodoxine)	Meat and poultry, fish, bananas, whole grain cereals, dairy products	Cervical abnormalities and cancer, diabetes
Vitamin B_{12} (Cyanocobalamin)	Fish, poultry, eggs, and milk, B_{12} enriched soy produce (no vegetable contains B_{12})	Anxiety, depression, mood swings, fatigue
Vitamin C (Ascorbic acid)	Citrus fruits, strawberries, broccoli, green peppers	Excessive menstrual bleeding, cervical abnormalities and cancer, chloasma
Vitamin D (Calciferol)	Sunlight, oily fish, fortified cereals and bread, fortified margarine	Poor calcium absorption, leading to an increase in the risk of osteoporosis
Vitamin E (Tocopherol)	Vegetable oils, green leafy vegetables, cereals, dried beans, whole grains, bread	Hot flashes, anxiety, vaginal problems (e.g. dryness), hypothyroidism, chloasma, atherosclerosis, osteoarthritis, fibrocystic breast disease

menopause, but this has not been medically verified. It may also relieve vaginal dryness when applied as an oil directly to the vagina as well as when it is taken in the diet.

CALCIUM

Experts recommend that women over 40 should take the equivalent of 1,500 mg of calcium a day (1,000 mg if they are on HRT), and women over 60 should take 1,200 mg. Calcium is essential for long-term bone health to protect you against osteoporosis (see p. 28); it will also protect your heart and lower blood fats.

Calcium absorption There is a misconception that in order to increase your daily calcium intake you can simply take calcium tablets. Unfortunately, taken on their own, these are difficult to absorb, and the calcium that is absorbed cannot be utilized by the bones and is excreted in the urine. To maximize the effect of calcium supplements, it is essential that both estrogen and small amounts of vitamin D are present.

Calcium supplements If you think you need a calcium supplement, seek medical advice. There are many types on the market, and deciding which one to use is a decision you should reach with your doctor. Different tablets are derived from different sources, and some are combined with other nutrients for better absorption or because the nutrients work as a unit within the body.

Calcium and phosphorus Taken correctly, phosphorus will enhance the amount of calcium absorbed by the bones. The diet of most people is too high in phosphorus, adversely affecting retention of calcium. To reestablish the correct ratio, reduce your intake of high-phosphorus foods drastically. This means eliminating processed foods such as canned meats, instant soups, and soft drinks, which offer little nutrition. Check food labels and avoid those that contain sodium phosphate, potassium phosphate, phosphoric acid, pyrophosphate, or polyphosphate.

OTHER BENEFICIAL MINERALS

Magnesium is instrumental in keeping calcium soluble in the bloodstream and may also help if you have low energy and a lack of vitality. A magnesium deficiency disturbs the

ACHIEVING A HEALTHIER DIET

The following simple guidelines may make it easier to change your eating patterns.

- *Keep your meals simple and easy. Cut down preparation time.*

- *Eat the largest meal of the day early; have a hearty breakfast, a light lunch, and an even lighter dinner.*

- *Eat a variety of foods so that you get a range of nutrients; don't eat the same foods every day out of habit.*

- *Make the transition to raw, high-fiber food slowly. Don't worry if it takes a few months to change your dietary habits.*

- *Identify any "high stress" foods and start substituting these with low stress ones (see p. 55).*

calcification of bone, impairs bone growth, and reduces calcium levels. Diets deficient in magnesium may lead to skeletal abnormalities including osteoporosis (see p. 28). Potassium is essential for normal muscle contraction and heart function; zinc is needed for hormone and brain function, and for building new cells. Fortunately, many foods contain magnesium, potassium, and zinc together.

MINERALS THAT WILL BENEFIT MENOPAUSAL COMPLAINTS

MINERAL	SOURCE	COMPLAINT
Calcium	Milk and milk products, dark-green leafy vegetables, citrus fruits, dried peas, and beans	Osteoporosis, hyperlipidemia (high concentration of blood fat), hypertension (high blood pressure)
Magnesium	Green leafy vegetables, nuts, soybeans, whole grain cereals	Osteoporosis, fatigue, diabetes, coronary artery disease, anxiety, depression
Potassium	Orange juice, bananas, dried fruits, peanut butter, meat	Fatigue, heart disease, hypertension (high blood pressure), anxiety, depression
Zinc	Meat, liver, eggs, poultry, seafood	Osteoporosis
Iron	Nuts, liver, red meats, egg yolk, green leafy vegetables, dried fruits	Anemia caused by excessive menstrual bleeding
Iodine	Seafood, fish, seaweed	Hypothyroidism, fibrocystic breast disease
Chromium	Meat, cheese, whole grains, breads	Hypoglycemia (low blood sugar)
Selenium	Seafood, meat, whole grain cereals	Fibrocystic breast disease, breast cancer
Manganese	Nuts, fruits, and vegetables, whole grain cereals	Atherosclerosis
Bioflavonoids	All citrus fruits, especially their pulp and pith	Hot flashes, excessive menstrual bleeding, vaginal problems, anxiety, irritability, and other emotional problems

You require magnesium for the efficient absorption of calcium, vitamin D, and phosphorus, thus emphasizing the importance of nutrient interrelationships. Recent evidence suggests that the balance between calcium and magnesium is an especially important one. If the calcium level is raised magnesium intake needs to be increased as well. The optimum calcium/magnesium ratio is two to one. So, if you are taking 1,000 mg of calcium, you will need to take 500 mg of magnesium to maintain a balance.

FIBER

Roughage is a particularly important part of any healthy diet. It keeps your gut healthy and promotes regular bowel movements, which helps prevent the distension and bloating that many women experience during menopause. It also helps bowel conditions such as irritable bowel syndrome and diverticulitis. Fiber can also give you a feeling of fullness and satisfaction that helps you to control your appetite, combat cravings, and avoid binges. There is good evidence to show that a woman who eats a high-fiber diet is less likely to suffer from a variety of cancers, including cancer of the colon and breast cancer. It may also protect against heart disease. Foods that are rich in fiber include whole grains (brown rice, whole meal pasta), dark-green leafy vegetables (collard greens, spinach), legumes (peas, beans, lentils), cereals, and nuts such as peanuts and cashews. See right for easy ways to increase the fiber content of your diet.

WATER

Water is a much neglected dietary element that is particularly important during menopause. It performs a wide range of functions in the body: it acts as a solvent for nutrients, oxygen, hormones, antibodies, and waste products; it helps to eliminate waste from the body as urine; it keeps both the skin and the mucous membranes plump and moist; and it lubricates the joints.

Water leaves the body in the form of urine and feces; it is also expired as water vapor and perspired as sweat. It serves as the body's natural radiator, keeping the skin cool. When perspiration evaporates from the surface of the skin, it turns into water vapor, using the body's internal heat to do so.

INCREASING FIBER

The following simple ways will help you increase your fiber intake.

- *Switch to high-fiber bread.*

- *Have high-fiber cereal for your breakfast.*

- *Eat high-fiber soups – such as bean, lentil, or corn.*

- *Use different types of beans and peas in your green salads.*

- *Use dark-green salad leaves, such as spinach, arugula, and endive, instead of pale iceberg lettuce.*

- *Eat bean dips with raw vegetables or whole-wheat pita bread.*

- *Use unbleached flour, nuts, and sesame seeds in your standard recipes, where appropriate.*

- *Snack on whole grain crackers and dried fruits.*

- *Eat muffins instead of cakes and cookies.*

REDUCING SUGAR

Most people eat too much sugar – follow the guidelines below to cut down.

• *Reduce your intake of convenience foods, relishes, ketchup, cakes, cookies, candy, and carbonated drinks, all of which have high levels of sugar.*

• *Avoid refined carbohydrate foods such as white flour, white bread, white sugar, or white rice, which are low in fiber and can contribute to obesity.*

• *When cooking, try to cut the amount of sugar in a recipe by about one-third; this won't spoil the taste at all.*

• *Satisfy cravings for chocolate and other sweet foods with healthier sweet alternatives, such as fresh fruit and fruit juice.*

• *Eat more fiber. A high-fiber diet will fill you up so that you are less likely to want a snack.*

• *If you have a sweet tooth, substitute a healthier sweetener, such as honey, which also has a sweeter taste, weight for weight. You can also have fruit rather than eating sweet pastries, cakes, and cookies.*

• *Use artificial sweeteners to sweeten without adding calories.*

• *Replace chocolate and cocoa with carob. It tastes similar to chocolate but is better for you and can control a sugar craving. Unfortunately, it is high in fat and should only be eaten occasionally.*

On average, we need four to six pints (two to three liters) of fluid every day simply to replace the amount we lose. Half of what we need comes from food, in the form of fruits and vegetables; the other half must come from drinking – about six to eight glasses a day. Any fluid is better than no fluid, but pure water is best, followed by fresh fruit juices and low-fat milk. Beverages containing caffeine or alcohol are not such good choices because they are diuretic and increase the amount of water we lose. Drinks containing lots of sugar are fattening and bad for the teeth.

BAD FOODS

There are two food groups that are detrimental to menopausal women: "nonfoods," such as sugar, that are high in calories but low in nutrients; and highly processed prepared foods that are nutritionally inferior and don't contain the mysterious micronutrients, enzymes, and trace elements that are found in natural foods. Many prepared foods contain salt, and blood pressure, bloating, and fluid retention are all adversely affected by salt. See p. 55 for ways of reducing your salt intake.

There are also foods and substances that can be described as "nutrient depleters" because they diminish the effect of many healthy foods. Nutrient depleters include alcohol, cigarettes, caffeine, and some medicines such as barbiturates, cortisone (an antirheumatic medication), laxatives, and diuretics. For instance, vitamin A is lost by coffee, alcohol, and processed foods; vitamin E is depleted by smoking cigarettes and from polyunsaturated fats through freezing; vitamin B is depleted by sugar, processed foods, dieting, coffee, and tea, and also by taking some medicines, such as cortisone and antacids; calcium by sugar, fat, and spinach; and potassium by fasting, salt, and coffee. Try to keep your intake of nutrient depleters low.

FAT

Most of us consume nearly half our calories in fat, and much of this comes in the form of saturated fat, that is, from dairy products such as cheese, butter and cream, and meat such as beef, lamb, and pork. It is also found in many processed and canned foods. Saturated fat can be particularly dangerous for menopausal women because a high intake is directly linked to cancers, heart disease, strokes, high blood pressure, and obesity, and, because of lowering levels of estrogen, women are becoming more vulnerable to these diseases at this point in their lives. However, polyunsaturated fats, such as those found in certain vegetable and fish oils, can help remove cholesterol from the tissues and protect the heart against heart disease.

To obtain essential fats and oils, eat raw seeds and nuts sparingly. Cook with vegetable oils such as corn, olive, sunflower, soybean, or safflower. Eat low-fat dairy products such as skimmed milk, and substitute plain yogurt for cream in desserts and main dishes. Cut down the amount of cheese you use when cooking so that it becomes a garnish rather than a main ingredient. Alternatively, replace cheese with tofu, which is high in calcium. You can also replace milk in recipes with soy milk.

HIGH-STRESS FOODS

These are substances, such as sugar, caffeine, and alcohol, that contribute to various menopausal problems. High-stress foods such as those listed below contain few nutrients and, in some cases, they may be addictive. In addition, avoid black pepper, monosodium glutamate (MSG), and very hot spices (which often worsen hot flashes), or cut the amount in half.

REDUCING SALT

Follow the guidelines below to cut back your salt consumption.

- *Cut down on prepared foods, such as hamburgers, salad dressings, hot dogs, pizzas, and French fries. If you're buying these foods, always look for brands that have no added salt.*

- *Avoid adding salt to already-cooked food. Fruits, vegetables, meat, and grains contain all the salt you will ever need.*

- *Enhance natural salt in foods by using flavorings such as garlic, herbs, spices, and lemon.*

- *Substitute potassium-based salt for table salt – it's healthy and doesn't exacerbate high blood pressure or heart disease.*

SUBSTITUTES FOR HIGH-STRESS FOODS	
HIGH-STRESS FOOD	SUBSTITUTES
1 cup (4 oz) white flour	1 cup (4 oz) whole-wheat flour
1 square chocolate	1 square of carob or 1 tablespoon powdered carob
1 tablespoon coffee	1 tablespoon decaffeinated coffee
½ teaspoon salt	½ teaspoon of one of the following: potassium salt substitute, yeast extract, basil, tarragon, oregano
4 fl oz (125 ml) wine	4 fl oz (125 ml) low-alcohol wine
8 fl oz (250 ml) beer	8 fl oz (250 ml) low-alcohol beer
8 fl oz (250 ml) milk	8 fl oz (250 ml) soy milk
¾ cup (5 oz) sugar	One of the following: ¼ cup molasses, ½ cup honey, ½ cup maple syrup, ½ cup barley malt, 2 cups apple juice

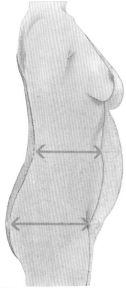

CHANGING SHAPE

KEY

↔ Premenopausal figure: waist smaller than hips, healthy pattern.

↔ Postmenopausal figure: waist larger than hips, high-risk pattern.

Obesity and risk
The pattern of obesity is important in determining risk, with deposits of fat on the waist and stomach conferring a higher risk than fat on the hips and thighs. This pattern is characteristic of postmenopausal women and is also related to an increased risk of heart disease.

WEIGHT CONTROL

Being too thin at any time of life is unhealthy. Some fat is essential for good health, and this is never more true than at menopause. We now know that women are healthier after menopause if they are 13–18 lb (6–8 kg) heavier than they were before. If you were not overweight before menopause, therefore, and providing your weight gain during and after stays within this figure, your extra pounds should not affect your health. If you have gained more than this, however, and if your waist-to-hip ratio is higher than 0.8 (see p. 24), you should take steps to control your weight. Obesity is potentially dangerous and it can make you more susceptible to heart disease and high blood pressure, among other conditions.

Weight increase is gradual in both men and women as they age, but for women it may become especially noticeable during menopausal and postmenopausal years. There are at least two factors involved here. First, lack of estrogen leads to changes in body shape and fat distribution so that the waist thickens and fat is deposited on the front of the abdomen. Second, our metabolic rate slows down as we mature and, by about the age of 55, we need fewer calories. Unless we have a regular and frequent exercise regime incorporated into our lives, continuing to eat at our usual rate will lead inexorably to weight gain.

POSITIVE EATING PATTERNS

Although you need fewer calories at this time of your life, your body's nutritional needs remain the same. Calorie-counting may be too time-consuming for anyone to maintain in the long term; it's much better to concentrate on having a diet that is well-balanced and contains no "empty" high-calorie foods such as sugar and fat. It's within your power to change not only what you eat but how you eat. Eating five or even six small meals at regular intervals, for instance, is very effective in terms of weight control. Each time you eat you use energy for digestion, and, if you eat very small quantities, the amount of energy expended in digestion can help compensate for the energy absorbed from the food. Small, frequent meals also prevent blood sugar levels from dropping, which can be accompanied by cravings for food.

Many studies have been carried out to show the differences between people who eat small, frequent meals and those who eat fewer, larger ones. The latter invariably have more body fat than the former. Some dieters find that a diet based on a nibbling pattern helps prevent hunger pangs, and there is some evidence that this may speed up weight loss. Your digestive system probably prefers a nibbling pattern diet, particularly if you suffer from indigestion or peptic ulcers.

Try not to go on crash diets or long-term diets that are little more than starvation. The initial weight loss may be impressive, but less than half of this will be fat; most will be water, and it could include some of your precious body protein. A diet that restricts total caloric intake to under a thousand calories is only just adequate. Very strict diets, those around 500 calories, cannot provide all the required nutrients for an adult woman.

The attraction of a crash diet is that it offers severely obese people a chance to lose up to about three to six pounds (one to two kilograms) per week. However, there is a great deal of research to show that toward the end of a long period of this kind of dieting, the rate of weight loss decelerates and the weight starts to be gained back when normal eating patterns are resumed. In other words, the body adapts to starvation.

The fewer calories we give the body, the less it needs, until it can finally get by on less than 300 a day. A return to normal eating will cause an inevitable increase in weight as body stores of glycogen are replaced – extremely depressing if you have made a great effort to shed excess weight. It is common for a person coming off a starvation diet to go on eating binges and find herself on a treadmill of intermittent starving and bingeing that is extremely damaging to her health and self-image.

CHANGING MEAL PATTERNS

Rather than having a set menu for breakfast, lunch, and dinner, think in terms of what type of food you would like to eat and how much time and energy you have to prepare it. For example, choose to cook a more elaborate meat meal over the weekend when you have plenty of time both to prepare and eat, and a nutritious but simple-to-make soup or pasta meal for weekdays, when you have less energy to devote to either.

WATCHING YOUR WEIGHT

Try the following tips to help curb your appetite.

- *Drink 8 fl oz of water before you start to eat. This will make you feel more satiated at the end of a meal.*

- *Put your food on a small plate. This controls the amount you can reasonably eat at one sitting.*

- *The more time you take eating food, the more satisfied you're likely to feel. People who overeat usually eat quickly and have to eat more in order to feel satisfied.*

- *Exercising an hour or so before a meal can help suppress your appetite.*

- *Eat your largest meal early in the day, when you have more time to burn up the calories you've eaten. Avoid eating large meals late in the evening – sleeping during the night does not burn off very many calories.*

Although many of us don't do enough exercise, a small percentage of women become psychologically addicted to exercise, experiencing the need to train every day, and feeling guilty if they miss a single session.

• *If you are addicted to exercise, don't be afraid that if you stop, even for a while, you will become unfit and overweight. This is untrue. Even competitive athletes have breaks in which they train lightly or not at all.*

• *If you feel your need to exercise is compulsive, or if it is accompanied by anxiety and depression, seek medical help.*

KEEPING FIT

Without doubt, exercise is the menopausal woman's best friend – it allows you to control your body and emotions by using your internal resources. Each time you exercise, your adrenal glands are stimulated to convert the male hormone androstenedione into estrogen. A minimum of four 30-minute exercise sessions each week will be enough to keep you supplied with estrogen. As you become older, your cardiorespiratory fitness, your strength, and your flexibility all begin to decline. For people who remain active, however, all of these things decrease at a lower rate than in those who become inactive (an average of 5 percent per decade after the age of about 20, as opposed to 9 percent per decade).

Long-term exercise also means that you will have stronger bones and a lower risk of osteoporosis than nonexercisers. Although every woman is different, most of us lose 25–35 percent of our bone mass by the time we reach the age of 65. Bone loss begins around the age of 35, proceeds slowly up to menopause, then accelerates during the five to seven years after menopause, when estrogen levels are low.

Women who do weight-bearing exercises, such as low-impact aerobics, walking, running, or weight training in their 20s and 30s can increase their bone density before loss sets in. Beginning exercise later in life can restore small amounts – about 4 percent. Unfortunately, you cannot "store" the benefits of exercise; it must be ongoing to confer its many benefits.

EXERCISE AS A MENTAL TONIC

Regular exercise may also have a significant effect on our mental agility by increasing the amount of oxygen supplied to the brain. In a recent comparison between sedentary older women and older women who exercised regularly, after four months the latter group processed information faster in tests.

Apart from increasing the oxygen supply to the brain, exercise may also slow down the loss of dopamine in the brain. Dopamine is a neurotransmitter that helps to prevent the shaking and stiffness that can come with old age (a severe shortage of it results in the exaggerated tremors of Parkinson's disease). Since exercise can slow down dopamine loss, it is therefore particularly beneficial as we grow older. Exercise can also prevent our reaction times from slowing down.

THE BENEFITS OF REGULAR EXERCISE

- A reduced risk of heart disease.
- A lower chance of developing diabetes.
- Maintenance of muscle strength.
- Higher levels of the healthy type of cholesterol in the blood.
- Healthier bones and less chance of developing osteoporosis later in life.
- A more efficient immune system.
- Reduced body fat.
- Better appetite control.
- Increased mental agility.
- Fewer headaches.
- Improved sleep quality.
- Flexible joints.

The type of exercise you do obviously depends largely on resources, how much time is available, and your own personal preferences. Today there is a wide range of opportunities available, and not only in sports centers, health clubs, and fitness classes. If you need or prefer to exercise in your own home, you will find some basic effective exercises to preserve muscle strength and tone on the following pages. And there are also many excellent exercise videos and other publications on this subject on the market.

You may prefer a sport such as tennis, bowling, or squash, all of which offer the added attraction of meeting and socializing with people. Likewise, joining any aerobics or exercise class can provide a social aspect that may encourage you to exercise more regularly. Less rigorous and more traditional forms of exercise such as walking and swimming also offer viable alternatives, and keep the body fit and supple.

Recently, there has been a move away from aerobics toward strength training and weight-bearing exercise. Recent research suggests that any exercise involving weights can delay loss of bone and muscle tissue, a natural consequence of aging. Weight-bearing exercise also helps the flow of sugar from the blood into muscle tissue, which may lower the risk of diabetes and heart disease.

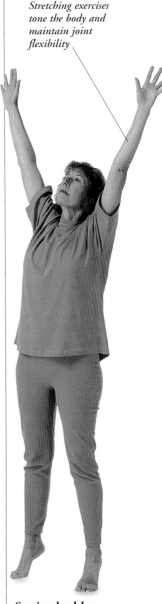

Stretching exercises tone the body and maintain joint flexibility

Staying healthy
Exercise not only increases your physical fitness and resistance to disease, it also has an uplifting effect on your mood.

GENERAL EXERCISES

These exercises encourage
mobility and preserve muscle
strength and tone. Try to do
each set at least 10 times a day.

UPPER BODY EXERCISES

These promote flexibility of the shoulders,
neck, and back, and alleviate problems
such as headaches and painfully knotted
muscles in the neck and back. They
also improve your posture.

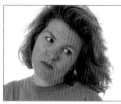

Head rolls
Starting with your chin
on your chest, slowly
roll your head around
to your right shoulder.
Hold this position and
then slowly roll your
head back, and around
to your left shoulder.

**Throwing off back and
shoulder tension**
Let your arms hang loosely by
your sides, and let your head
drop forward. Throw your
right hand over your left
shoulder as if you have a ball
in your hand. Repeat this on
the other side.

*Lean back
simultaneously with
your weight evenly
balanced*

**Hanging back in
a circle**
Make a circle, hold hands
with the person next to
you, and lean backward.
If you do this with a
mirror behind you, bend
back so you can see your
face in it. You can do this
with one other partner.

FEET AND LEG MOVEMENTS

Maintaining mobility
and flexibility in your
feet and weight-bearing
joints is important as you
get older, since it will help
prevent debilitating
physical conditions such
as arthritis.

Kicking your boots off
Kicks not only increase
articulation in the knees and
hips, they also relieve anger
and tension. Support yourself
by holding onto a door frame
and kick forward, as if you
were kicking off shoes. Do this
several times with each leg.

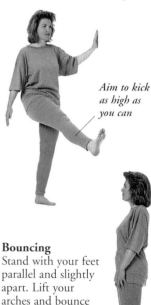

*Aim to kick
as high as
you can*

Bouncing
Stand with your feet
parallel and slightly
apart. Lift your
arches and bounce
gently up and down
without bending your
knees. This improves
strength and
flexibility in your
feet and calves.

Knee moves

Lie on your back, raise your right knee, and place your left palm on your right kneecap. Gently bend and stretch your leg. Now move your foot around and around in a circle, keeping your knee still. Repeat with the other knee.

Move your leg slowly, drawing as big a circle as you can with your foot

Stepping up and down

Stand on a soft mat with your feet slightly apart and kneel down on your right knee, followed by the other knee. Now, leading with your right foot, and keeping your spine vertical, go back to a standing position. Repeat until your thigh muscle gets tired and then repeat with your left leg. This is the way that you should stand up after you have been sitting or working on the floor.

Your back should be straight as you come up from the floor

Squats

Resting in a squatting position increases flexibility in your knees and calves, and strengthens your thigh muscles. Make sure that your feet are parallel and that your knees are on either side of your body. If you cannot stay in a squatting position, hold onto a table leg to stop yourself falling backward.

Put your arms out in front of you to help balance yourself

Ankle moves

Sit on the floor with your legs straight, and support yourself with your arms behind you. Flex and point your feet as many times as feels comfortable. Now slowly rotate your ankles, first clockwise and then counterclockwise. This loosens joints and discourages puffiness.

Rest your weight on your hands or lean against a wall

Keep your feet flat to stretch your hamstrings

61

WAIST, HIPS, STOMACH, AND BOTTOM EXERCISES

After menopause, fat distribution changes so that more fat is on the waist and abdomen. These movements help to keep your abdominal muscles toned and your hip joints loose and flexible.

Move your knees slowly in an arc across your body to the left

Spinning top
Following the four steps on the right, kneel on the floor and shift your weight onto your bottom on the right-hand side of you. Bring your knees up and over onto the left side. Return to a kneeling position, then lift up your bottom and sit on the right-hand side again. If you repeat this movement, lifting your bottom over your feet, you should move around in a complete circle. You may need to use your hands to help you at first.

Pull your stomach muscles in

Make your movements smooth and fluid

Rest your weight on your right thigh

Full hip circling
Following the three steps on the right, lie on your back on the floor and slowly bring your right knee over to touch the floor on the left side of your body. Bring your right knee up toward your chest and hug it with your arms. Lower your bended leg to the floor, keeping it at right angles to your hip. Now slide the leg back into the original resting position. Repeat with the left leg.

Your arms should be above your head

Keep your thigh at right angles to your body

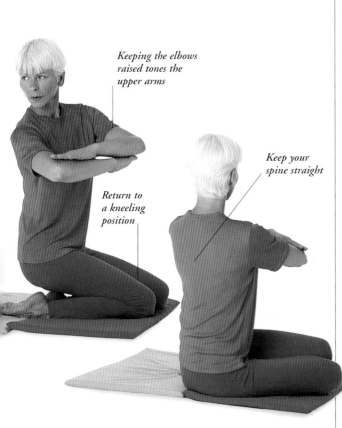

Keeping the elbows raised tones the upper arms

Return to a kneeling position

Keep your spine straight

Bottom and thigh toner
This exercise is so simple it doesn't require an illustration. Lie on your front and cross your ankles. Keeping your knees straight, raise both your legs a short distance off the ground and hold them there for a count of ten. Now cross your legs in the other direction and repeat. (Avoid this exercise if you suffer from back pain.)

Bottom racing
Practicing this simple exercise regularly will keep your buttocks toned. Sit with your legs straight out in front of you and move forward on your buttocks as fast as you can. Keep your arms stretched out straight in front of you.

Standing spiral twists
This straightforward exercise will help keep your spine supple. Stand with your feet apart, your arms loosely by your sides, and twist at the waist as far as you can. Now twist in the other direction and increase your momentum. Let your arms swing under their own gravity.

Clasp your knee as close to your chest as you can

Try to make your knee touch the ground when you lower your leg

Use your hand to push your knee down gently

Support your head on a cushion

63

CONTROLLING
SMOKING

Try the following to reduce nicotine intake.

• *Smoke less than five cigarettes a day.*

• *Always throw away a long stub.*

• *Don't inhale.*

• *Always smoke low-tar cigarettes.*

• *Always smoke filter-tip cigarettes.*

• *Keep cigarettes as far away from you as possible, so that getting one involves the maximum effort.*

ABANDONING BAD HABITS

Maintaining optimum health depends not only on adopting good habits but also on abandoning bad ones. For example, even if you eat the recommended daily amount of calcium and vitamin C, if you are a smoker this amount will not be sufficient, since smoking depletes essential vitamins and minerals.

SMOKING

It has been proved that inhaling cigarette smoke causes lung cancer, bronchitis, and heart disease. For women of any age, it is bad for your health, and it speeds up aging of the skin. If you are still smoking, it is particularly important that you stop before menopause. Smokers reach menopause up to five years earlier than nonsmokers (this includes passive smokers). Hot flashes tend to be more troublesome; smokers are more likely to get osteoporosis; and smokers are also more likely to have a heart attack.

Giving up smoking is difficult and some people only succeed when they have a dramatic health reason: menopause, in my opinion, is a dramatic health reason. If you really find it impossible to give up completely, try to follow the controlling tips on the left.

ALCOHOL

Although drinking can have a relaxing effect, hot flashes can be triggered by alcohol, and, for this reason alone, you should keep a careful eye on your intake.

A woman's response to alcohol differs according to the point she is at in her menstrual cycle: drink for drink, she will have higher alcohol levels during the premenstrual and ovulatory phases than at other times of the month. A woman's body contains 5–10 percent less water than a man's, so the same amount of alcohol will be more concentrated in her system and thus have a greater toxic effect on the body. Consequently, it takes less alcohol, consumed over fewer years, to cause liver damage in women than men.

Excessive drinking usually has a psychological origin, and menopausal women may be more vulnerable to alcoholism, especially if they feel that their former role is being eroded. We may also drink heavily if we are bored or unfulfilled. Understanding why we drink heavily is the first step to overcoming the problem.

Alcohol consumption is measured in units per week. Fourteen units per week is considered the healthy amount for a woman to drink. Half a pint of beer, an ounce of hard liquor, or a glass of wine is one unit. A light drinker would drink one to five units per week, and a moderate drinker 6–14 units. If you drink more than 14 units a week, you could be damaging your health, and if you drink more than 21, you may be on the verge of alcoholism. If the latter applies to you, or if you feel that your drinking is becoming a problem, you should seek medical help.

Menopausal women have acute reasons for limiting alcohol intake. Alcohol is an antinutrient, depleting the body of vitamins A, B, and C, and it is a powerful oxidant and can lead to premature wrinkling of the skin.

CAFFEINE

Caffeine is a powerful drug that has a stimulating effect on the brain and a diuretic effect on the kidneys – it increases the amount of urine you pass. Although caffeine is present in the greatest quantity in coffee, it is also contained in some medications and in tea, chocolate, and cola drinks. It can be a pick-me-up and, in small doses, may result in clearer thinking and sharper awareness. Larger doses, however, can give you "coffee nerves" – an anxious, fluttery feeling.

Caffeine can be particularly bad for menopausal women because it can actually trigger a hot flash. It also causes a temporary rise in blood pressure. If you have a weight problem, you should monitor your caffeine intake carefully, since too much can encourage the pancreas to release more insulin. This lowers your blood sugar, making you hungry and therefore inclined to binge.

Trying to cut out caffeine from your diet in one fell swoop may bring on withdrawal symptoms. Reduce your intake gradually, make sure your diet is rich in fiber, and drink plenty of water.

One way to reduce your consumption is to use a mixture of regular and decaffeinated coffee, gradually increasing the amount of the latter until the caffeine part is replaced. You can also substitute herbal teas, but check out the ingredients, since some herbal teas contain caffeine.

CONTROLLING YOUR ALCOHOL INTAKE

Try the following to reduce your alcohol intake.

- *Try to drink an equal quantity of water with alcohol.*

- *Eliminate drinks before and after meals, such as aperitifs and liqueurs.*

- *Always eat when you drink.*

- *Offer friends more non-alcoholic drinks, and drink more of these yourself.*

- *Skip the occasional round of drinks.*

- *If you have been drinking during the evening, have some water before you go to bed; put a full glass by your bedside in case you need a drink during the night.*

CARING FOR YOUR BODY

Keeping your body in good condition throughout the menopausal years requires the same combination of exercise, health-monitoring, and hygiene that it always has. However, you need to pay more attention to certain parts of the body such as teeth, eyes, ears, and legs.

EYES

Visual defects that occur with age usually result from the changing shape of the eye, rather than the impaired functioning of its various parts.

Presbyopia becomes quite common in middle age, and develops because the lens is less able to change its shape to focus on what you are looking at. As a result, vision becomes blurred. Your optician will fit you with inwardly curved (convex) lenses to increase the power of your own lens, so that objects focus on the retina.

The cells of the retina also become less sensitive to light as you grow older, and it can become more difficult to read or see when brightness levels are low. On average, an 85-year-old woman needs approximately eight times as much light as a young person in order to see as well. The lens can also become yellowish, which makes it difficult to distinguish between different colors. Blue and green are filtered out, but warm colors like red and orange are easier to see.

Even if you think your eyesight is perfectly all right, always make sure you have regular checkups because a variety of disorders, such as glaucoma or cataracts, are more common in older people.

EARS

By the age of 50, some of us will be less able to hear higher-pitched sounds, but most of us should be able to look forward to normal hearing beyond the age of 60. Hearing loss is usually due to changes in the inner ear.

As we get older, we tend to lose the fine hair cells within the cochlea (inner ear) that activate the neurons in the auditory nerve. This is the most common cause of hearing loss, one that cannot be helped by a hearing aid. If impairment is not due to damage to the auditory nerve or to the hair cells inside the cochlea, a hearing aid can make a big difference in the ability to cope.

The outer ear is rich in sebaceous glands that produce wax. Ear wax has several useful functions: it's an antiseptic and a lubricant, and it prevents foreign substances from reaching the eardrum and the middle ear. Daily washing is all that's needed to keep the outer ear clean. Wax should never be removed by cotton swabs – it will be driven down the ear canal where it will become impacted. It can then only be removed with warmed eardrops that dissolve the wax.

Even if you feel that both your ears and hearing are fine, always have regular checkups to make sure that they both remain healthy.

MOUTH

The mouth is kept clean and healthy by the acts of talking, eating, and drinking. Halitosis (bad breath) can be due to bad dental hygiene, mouth infection, dental decay, or smoking. Regular tooth brushing is essential. Mouth washes and deodorant sprays do not compensate for bad hygiene and only cure bad breath temporarily.

By mid-adult life, most of us will have fillings, inlays, and crowns, and we may also have a bridge or partial denture. At menopause, the gums begin to recede due to lack of collagen, so the teeth become more exposed. Care of your mouth and teeth are as crucial now as they were when you were a child; follow the care tips on the right for optimum dental health.

Any sore patches on your tongue, gums, or the inside of your cheeks that last more than two weeks should be seen by your doctor or dentist. A dry mouth can be relieved by sucking a sugarless hard candy or having a drink of water. Always have the sharp edge of a tooth attended to by a dentist since it could cause an ulcer. Gum shrinkage that leads to loose dentures should also be treated.

GENITALS

The vagina is a self-cleansing organ that does not benefit from excessive cleansing; in fact, overzealous washing can upset the delicate bacterial balance necessary for vaginal health. It's far better to underclean than to overclean, and this applies to all parts of the body lined with delicate mucous membranes.

You should try to avoid using douches, antiseptics in the bath, and vaginal deodorants. Overuse can kill off bacteria that are the first line of defense against invaders

CARING FOR YOUR TEETH

Try the following simple guidelines to keep your teeth strong and healthy.

● *Keep plaque at bay by regular tooth brushing in the morning and at night, and after eating sweet foods. (Plaque causes tartar, which in turn can lead to pyorrhea, the worst enemy of middle-aged teeth and gums.)*

● *Take care to clean in between your teeth (we develop spaces between our teeth as we get older). Dental floss or a tiny brush with a specially designed handle is suitable.*

● *Take a toothbrush with you if you're eating out so that you can brush your teeth after your meal.*

● *Visit your dental hygienist every three months for plaque removal, and visit your dentist every six months for general checkups.*

such as *candida*, the fungus that causes thrush. The natural vaginal smell is preferable to an artificial perfume and it plays an important part in sexual attraction; you may be less attractive to your partner if you take pains to camouflage it.

Under ordinary circumstances, bathing daily is sufficient to keep your genitals clean, although in hot weather you may feel comfortable washing more frequently. When you are washing, try not to use soap inside the outer lips of the vulva. You can wash the anal area as much as you like – it will not be harmful – but the vulval area is much more delicate and you should treat it gently. Unless you are sweating profusely or having sex a great deal, never use soap and water more than twice a day, and always use a gentle soap. At other times, it's quite sufficient to use water alone. You can wet a couple of cotton balls in water and wipe once from the front to the back of the perineal area, then throw them away. If you can't wash yourself during the course of the day, use baby wipes after you've been to the bathroom, again from front to back, and using them only once before disposing of them.

LEGS AND FEET

To maintain an active lifestyle, we should pay special attention to our legs and feet. Hardening of the arteries and increasingly poor circulation can take their toll, especially on lower limbs and feet.

You'll avoid blisters and sore heels and toes if you wear comfortable, supple, low-heeled shoes most of the time. A shoe that fits well should grip your heel and instep, and not press on your toes. Whenever you can, sit with your feet up so that any fluid can drain away and the blood can flow more easily. This will also speed healing if you get any kind of cut, abrasion, or sore. As you get older, minor injuries take longer to heal, and this particularly applies to the feet. Treat cuts and sores promptly with a simple antiseptic cream and if they don't heal within a few days, consult your doctor. If you suffer from diabetes, consult your doctor immediately if you have a break in the skin of your legs and feet. Feet become more prone to infections with age, so never soak them in hot water – this makes the skin soggy so it is a perfect medium for bacteria. You should also avoid wearing tight pants or panty hose on your legs, since this will worsen circulation and hinder blood returning to the heart via the veins.

Chilblains tend to become more of a problem as you get older. You can help avoid them by keeping your feet warm and wearing thick, woolen socks or panty hose, and in cold weather, fleece-lined slippers and shoes. One way to discourage the development of chilblains is to start the day with a warm bath and massage your feet with lotion or oil, using circular movements, and then dry them with a rough towel. Never put your feet or legs near direct heat or hold them against a radiator.

Varicose veins are most often the result of deep vein thrombosis in the leg, and they run in families. See right for self-help measures if you suffer from them. Mild varicose veins can be injected so they shrink and eventually scar and shrivel. If they are extensive, they can be stripped out by a vascular surgeon. Modern surgery is less painful and requires less hospitalization than previously.

NAILS

Brittle and flaking nails can be a problem after menopause because waning estrogen levels result in poor quality collagen (see p. 16).

If your fingernails are brittle and flaky, avoid using nail polish remover, since this can dry them out even more. Use an emery board rather than scissors and metal files, and massage hand and nail cream into your cuticles daily. When you cut your toenails, use good-quality clippers and cut the nails straight across the top to the edges – never cut them steeply at the sides, since this encourages ingrown toenails. If your toenails are very thick, file them frequently and try to thin them down as well as shorten them. Trim both finger and toenails once a week to keep them in good condition. From menopause onward, it's wise to visit a podiatrist on a regular basis.

SKIN AND BLOOD VESSELS

Aging causes skin to become thinner and appear more transparent. Gradual changes to connective tissue are most easily seen on the backs of the hands, but are widespread throughout the body, resulting in conditions such as arthritis, hardening of the arteries, reduced lung capacity, and loss of skin tone.

CARING FOR VARICOSE VEINS

Try the following simple suggestions to make varicose veins more comfortable.

- *Wear support stockings or panty hose and avoid tight garters or bands.*

- *Keep your legs warm and moisturize them after washing.*

- *Try not to stand for long periods at a time.*

- *Rest legs in an upright position whenever possible; if you can, lie on the floor and put your legs up against the wall for 30 minutes before putting on support hose.*

- *Treat abrasions, bruises, or minor infections of the lower legs meticulously, and consult your doctor if necessary.*

CONTROLLING BLOOD PRESSURE

Follow the simple measures below to maintain your blood pressure at healthy levels.

• *Cut back on both smoking and alcohol use.*

• *Control your weight (see p. 57 for some self-help tips).*

• *Try relaxation and meditation exercises to reduce stress (see pp. 42–43); stress is another cause of high blood pressure.*

BLOOD PRESSURE

Some self-regulating mechanisms are lost as we age, such as the maintenance of blood pressure during changes in posture. This may result in dizziness, and a tendency to lose your balance when you have to get up suddenly, especially from a horizontal position. High blood pressure can, in fact, become an increasing hazard with age and can lead to serious health problems such as stroke and heart disease. Try to keep your blood pressure at a sensible level by following the simple guidelines outlined on the left.

LUNGS AND KIDNEYS

Cells in the lungs may be affected by age or disease. There is a decrease in the surface area of the air sacs, which can account for the breathlessness you may experience on exertion. Medically supervised exercise can play an important part in combating this problem.

Kidneys are affected by the deterioration of the circulatory system. The rate at which blood is filtered slows down and valuable minerals are reabsorbed more slowly. To keep your kidneys functioning properly, drink plenty of water, follow a healthy diet (see pp. 48–55), and exercise reasonably (see pp. 58–63).

BRAIN AND MIND

Because brain cells do not reproduce themselves, their function and number decrease as we grow older. The result of this is most apparent when it comes to memory, particularly when committing new experiences to memory. Opinions and attitudes can also become more rigid, so the acceptance of new ideas can become progressively more difficult. However, as long as mental skills are exercised continuously, they should not decline to any significant degree.

Although intellectual deterioration is considered to be a result of aging, it is actually a physical process that begins around the age of 16. For most of our adult lives, we do not notice any deterioration, mainly because we gain new experiences and knowledge, which compensate. This is why an alert mind coupled with a willingness to embrace new ideas, opinions, and situations will keep us mentally healthy. Just as an unused muscle wastes away, so does an unused mind.

NATURAL THERAPIES

Although many women seek medical help during their menopausal years, there are many strategies that you can adopt by yourself to manage your own treatment, including a range of natural therapies, from aromatherapy to yoga. All therapies have their strengths and weaknesses and most are better for some things than for others. Some you can practice yourself, while for others you will need to find a qualified practitioner in order to benefit from it. Knowledge is the key – and the information in this chapter will enable you to take the most appropriate course of action for yourself.

PRACTICING NATUROPATHY

Naturopaths consider nutrition to be the anchor of health, and treatment will usually involve fasting (one of the oldest therapeutic methods known). You will also be advised to:

• *Drink pure water.*

• *Eat organically grown, unprocessed and, as far as possible, uncooked food.*

• *Use food supplements from natural sources rather than vitamin supplements. Wheatgerm oil, kelp, and royal jelly can be particularly beneficial during menopause.*

• *Animal protein should not make up more than 25 percent of the diet.*

COMPLEMENTARY THERAPIES

Any medicine that heals or relieves discomfort without any harmful side effects is, in my opinion, good medicine. Although hormone replacement therapy is the major treatment advocated by the medical establishment, complementary practices offer many natural alternatives.

Traditional medicine is based on allopathy, a doctrine that follows the principle that when the working of the body goes wrong, the symptoms should be counteracted. An example of this practice would be treating constipation with a laxative.

In contrast to this approach, the major branches of complementary medicine argue that each body has a life force that becomes disturbed when that body becomes diseased but reasserts itself if the body stops being abused and is nourished correctly.

Just like the best traditional medicine, the best complementary medicine is holistic – it treats the whole person, rather than an isolated symptom. The true naturopath is skeptical of symptomatic remedies because they fail to treat the root cause of the illness.

NATUROPATHY

Many types of complementary medicine are based on naturopathy. Its principles are as follows:

• The patient is treated, not the disease.
• The whole body is treated, not just a part of it.
• The underlying factors causing the disease must be removed.
• Disease is a disturbance of a life force, demonstrated by tension, rigidity, or congestion somewhere in the body.
• The patient's own life force is the true healer.
• The body must have a "healing crisis" in which the life force cleanses the body by eliminating accumulated toxins. The use of drugs in orthodox medicine, while superficially curing the disease, drives it deep within the body, leaving behind a chronic condition for the future.

Naturopaths believe that health depends on adopting a well-balanced attitude by practicing relaxation, yoga, meditation, and psychotherapy. Some also include hydrotherapy (see p. 77) in their treatment programs.

AROMATHERAPY

Although this is a fairly new addition to complementary medicine, its roots go back several centuries. Human beings have a highly developed sense of smell, and we can react to an odor within a split second. Babies bond with their mothers through scent, and lovers are attracted by each other's pheromones, or chemical secretions. Smells can be mood-enhancing and they may relieve pain and illness. Massage using essential oils is relaxing and enjoyable and beneficial in reducing many stress-related conditions.

The oil essences that are used in aromatherapy are pure distillations from plants, and are very concentrated. In a dilute form, they can be inhaled and absorbed through the lining of the air passages. Essential oils can be used singly or blended, and they have different properties: some are antiviral, some affect blood pressure, and some are general healers.

Essential oils are absorbed through the skin during massage or bathing, and through the lungs when they are inhaled. Oral doses are not generally recommended except in the case of garlic, which may be taken in capsule form. The emphasis in aromatherapy is on the treatment of relatively minor ailments and the promotion of health and well-being, both physical and mental. For this reason, the use of essential oils has achieved a wide popularity in recent years.

USING ESSENTIAL OILS

Essential oils are very strong, so take care when using them. Try these simple tips.

- *Inhale as a vapor. Add three drops of essential oil to a bowl of steaming water, cover your head, and breathe in.*

- *Add a few drops to a warm bath. Spend at least 15 minutes in it to derive the full benefit.*

- *Apply to the skin as massage oil. Dilute with a base, such as sweet almond oil or soy oil. Add about 20 drops to 3.4 fl oz (100 ml) of base oil.*

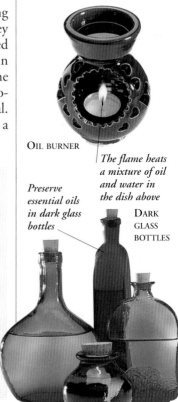

OIL BURNER

| *The flame heats a mixture of oil and water in the dish above*

Preserve essential oils in dark glass bottles

DARK GLASS BOTTLES

MENOPAUSAL REMEDIES

ESSENTIAL OIL	SYMPTOMS
Avocado, wheatgerm	Dry skin
Juniper, lavender, rosemary	Muscle and joint pain
Lavender, peppermint	Headaches
Basil	Fatigue
Neroli, lavender	Insomnia
Clary sage, rose	Depressed mood

USING HOMEOPATHIC REMEDIES

It's best to have a consultation to determine your constitutional "type," but if you treat yourself, bear in mind the following.

• *Increase the potency or seek medical advice if your symptoms are not relieved after six doses.*

• *Avoid substances such as coffee, peppermint, menthol, and camphor, which can counteract the effects of homeopathic remedies.*

• *Avoid homeopathic pills coated in lactose if you are allergic to milk.*

• *Take a remedy hourly if your symptoms are acute. For longer-term problems, remedies can be taken in the morning and at night.*

• *Stop taking a remedy as soon as your symptoms start to improve.*

• *Preserve remedies by storing them in a cool, dark place away from smells.*

HOMEOPATHY

This form of natural healing is based on the principle that a substance that produces the same symptoms as disease will, in a very dilute form, help to cure it. The venom of the bushmaster snake, lachesis, for instance, is very poisonous, but because it is used in such a dilute form, it is not toxic. The potency of remedies affects the efficacy of treatment – the more dilute the remedy, the greater the potency. Homeopathic remedies have a number after them that indicates how dilute they are. For instance, *pulsatilla 30* is more dilute and therefore more potent than *pulsatilla 6.*

The homeopathic view of menopausal problems is that they reflect existing imbalances, which can only be treated in relation to the mental and physical makeup of the individual. Women are encouraged to prepare for menopause by looking at their overall health and developing a positive attitude of self before its onset.

The emphasis upon the individual and her physical and emotional history, rather than the disorder she is suffering from, is fundamental to homeopathy. When consulting a homeopathic practitioner, your symptoms are assessed along with your personality and constitution, and likes and dislikes, to form the basis of your treatment. For example, the remedy *sepia* is suited to someone who is irritable, moody, or dejected.

If you would like to treat your symptoms homeopathically, it is very important to consult a qualified homeopathic practitioner.

MENOPAUSAL REMEDIES

REMEDY	SYMPTOMS
Lachesis	Hot flashes
Pulsatilla	Insomnia, PMS, joint pain
Sepia	Dry vagina, prolapse, flashes, thinning hair
Sulfur	Dry, itchy vulva and skin
Belladonna	Hot flashes and night sweats

HERBALISM

Some of the oldest methods of healing the sick are based on herbalism. Over the centuries, developments in orthodox medicine began to cast doubt on the efficacy of natural remedies, but since the 1950s herbalism has enjoyed renewed popularity. It can sometimes be compared favorably with modern drugs that may create allergies or spread resistant strains of bacteria.

Like homeopathy, the aims behind herbal treatment are to remove the cause of the symptoms rather than merely the symptoms themselves, and to improve the patient's general standard of health and well-being. A disadvantage of herbalism is that agreement over which remedies should be used for particular disorders is still surprisingly limited. However, it does offer an attractive alternative to other forms of conventional treatment in that it is based on natural principles and ingredients. Herbal remedies can also work as a complement to orthodox medicine.

Modern herbalism aims to correct what is wrong with the body by strengthening its natural functions so that it may heal itself. Herbs can be very effective in relieving menopausal symptoms, but although there is valuable anecdotal information about their benefits, few remedies have been subjected to tightly controlled clinical trials.

There are many herbs that can help to relieve both the physical and emotional symptoms of menopause, but there are three in particular that are associated with it: sage, agnus castus, and black cohosh.

Sage may help to alleviate hot flashes, and you can take it in tea form, made from fresh or dried sage. Simply pour boiling water onto two teaspoonfuls of leaves, infuse for ten minutes, and strain. Sage tea has quite a strong taste, and although some women find it calming, others find it unpalatable – if you don't like the taste, buy the herb in tablet form from a herbalist.

The herb agnus castus (also known as chaste tree) has long been associated with menopausal disorders, and it may help to normalize hormone levels, acting as a natural type of hormone replacement therapy. Some herbalists recommend the following combination of herbs to treat hot flashes: blackcurrant leaves, hawthorn tops, sage, and agnus castus. This may be drunk in an

USING HERBS

Follow these simple guidelines for effective herbal treatment.

● *Consult a qualified herbalist before taking herbs, especially if you have heart disease, high blood pressure, or glaucoma.*

● *Always use herbs in moderation, and, if possible, discuss dosage with a qualified herbalist before treatment.*

● *Discontinue use if you start to experience side effects.*

● *Give each herb a week or two to assess its efficacy.*

● *Don't take herbs for longer than a few months without a break.*

● *Check with your doctor before you take a herbal remedy if you are already taking medication.*

● *Don't put off seeking medical advice because you are taking a herbal remedy.*

● *Buy herbs from a reputable supplier because it is very easy to make mistakes in identification.*

infusion three times daily for six weeks. Black cohosh has estrogenic properties and can be of assistance if you are feeling weak and tense. It also has antispasmodic and sedative properties and will help alleviate premenstrual syndrome, pains, and bloating. Black cohosh works well in combination with agnus castus.

ACUPUNCTURE

The word acupuncture comes from the Latin and means "to pierce with a needle." The use of acupuncture in China has been widespread for 5,000 years, but it has only been acknowledged and practiced in the West during this century.

The theory behind acupuncture is that a life or energy force flows through the body along channels called meridians that are quite distinct from the lines followed by nerves. This life force must flow unimpeded if bodily health is to be maintained. When we get sick, the energy flowing along a particular meridian may be affected at a site considerably distant from the sick part of the body. The acupuncturist tries to restore the flow of energy in the affected meridian by using copper, silver, or gold needles inserted a small way into the flesh at specific points along the meridian. These needles are so fine that they can hardly be felt as they enter the skin. Depending on the position of the selected point, the needles may be inserted vertically, at an angle, or even sometimes almost horizontally. The needle is then rotated, moved up and down, or used to conduct heat or a mild electric current. This is thought to set up some kind of current along the meridian line. It passes to the central nervous system and has an effect on the organ or area that is malfunctioning by re-establishing the flow of energy through the meridian.

Acupuncture is one of the few Eastern medical practices that is widely accepted and used in the West, although its applications are not nearly as widespread here. In China, even major operations, including heart transplants and brain surgery, may be performed using acupuncture as the only form of general anesthetic.

The meridians
Acupuncture and acupressure are based on the theory that our life force flows along channels called meridians. When the flow of energy is disturbed, we get sick.

Acupressure points

Meridians

Electrical acupressure device
This handheld device is used to locate and apply pressure to the acupressure points.

ACUPRESSURE

This technique follows the same principles as acupuncture, but pressure, rather than needles, is applied to the energy meridians. Massaging the acupoints with the thumbs and fingers helps restore interrupted energy flow along the meridians. Pressure is applied to specific points, with the aim of stimulating the nerves that supply the affected organ.

Acupressure is claimed to help specific organs by releasing blocked energy. Unlike acupuncture, you can practice acupressure on yourself, although you may find it hard to locate the right pressure points at first. It can be used to alleviate pain, improve your general well-being, or target specific symptoms, such as joint stiffness.

HYDROTHERAPY

Hydrotherapy aims to increase the blood flow to the skin and eliminate toxins (this should be viewed with skepticism since they cannot be expelled through the skin – we have a liver to do that). It also draws blood and nourishment to internal organs then flushes it out again.

Most forms use hot and cold water alternately. The hot water dilates the blood vessels, increasing blood flow to the skin. This part of the treatment may last five, ten, or fifteen minutes, according to the severity of the condition and the patient's frailty. It should be avoided if you have any kind of heart condition since hydrotherapy can put an enormous strain on the heart. The second stage of therapy involves douching, sluicing, or showering in cold water, which causes the blood vessels to constrict, reducing blood flow and driving blood back to the heart and the purifying organs, such as the liver. Never take any of the treatments listed on the right without checking with your doctor first.

MASSAGE

Many claims are made about the virtues of massage – some are false, some plausible, and some indisputable. For example, massage does not help to break down fat, but it may relieve emotional tension, and it definitely speeds up local circulation and improves nourishment of tissues. During a massage, parts of the body are treated in a specific order. The direction of massage strokes is

WATER TREATMENTS

The following are the major therapeutic water treatments.

Sauna *Sitting in intense, dry heat is followed by a cold shower, then a second, shorter period in the sauna, followed by a scrub-down. It is said to improve circulation, tone up muscles, cleanse the skin, and create well-being.*

Scotch douche *Hot and cold water is sprayed alternately up and down the spine to stimulate the nerves. It is thought to relieve migraine.*

Sitz Bath *This is a two-section bath, one for hot water and one for cold. Your buttocks and hips sit in hot water for five to ten minutes while your feet are immersed in cold. You then switch around, with your feet in hot, body in cold. It flushes blood into the pelvic area to nourish it, then out again to carry off waste material.*

Steam Cabinets *This is like a traditional Turkish bath, except the head is outside the steam area. The heat is wet rather than dry, so it produces sweat faster. It is said to clear the skin of waste materials very efficiently. The body will feel very hot and some people may find it debilitating. After 15 minutes, the bather takes a cold shower to restore skin to normal. Treatment should be followed by rest.*

always toward the heart, assisting the return of blood to the heart to be oxygenated in the lungs. The patient lies down and the masseur massages each foot and leg in turn. Next comes the abdomen, followed by the fingers, hands, wrists, and arms, then the back of the body.

Swedish massage involves vigorous strokes, such as beating with the sides of the hands from the base of the spine to the neck and back again. Although it is usually a safe therapy, avoid vigorous massage if you have any sort of skin disease or if your skin has been injured.

Neuromuscular massage consists of pressing with the fingertips. Specific motor points in the muscles are deeply massaged in an attempt to diminish the output to the

TYPES OF MASSAGE STROKE

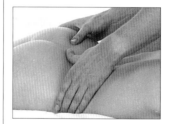

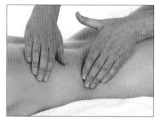

Pressing
Localized pressure can be given using the thumbs either in static form, pressing in one position, or circular, moving the thumbs in small circles.

Circling
This is a very simple stroke, in which you use the fingers and palms of both hands to massage the skin in firm, circular movements.

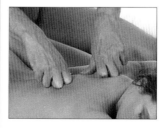

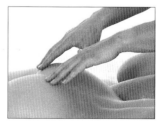

Knuckling
Here, the knuckles are used to exert pressure below the shoulder blades. This is good for getting rid of tension in painfully knotted muscles.

Feathering
This playful and gentle massage stroke involves lightly skimming the fingertips and fingernails across the surface of the skin.

sensory nerves to the area, and break the vicious circle of pain and muscle spasm from which we can suffer from time to time. Once muscular tension has been relieved using this technique, the muscle will be less likely to spring back into its previous tense position.

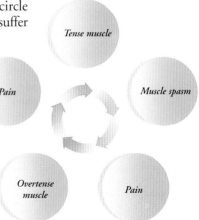

OSTEOPATHY

Modern osteopathy is based on the theory that our bodies have the ability to regulate and heal themselves, provided that they are structurally sound and nerve impulses and blood are able to move freely.

Harmful structural changes to the body may result from several things, including poor posture. Osteopathic stimulation tries to rectify these problems by manipulating the spinal vertebrae. Osteopaths also believe that relief of muscle spasm cures illnesses stemming from muscular strain.

Vicious circle of pain
Massage can relax the muscles and break the vicious circle of muscle tension and pain.

The two basic techniques of osteopathy are the massage of muscles in spasm and the manipulative correction of misaligned bones in the spinal column. This involves gentle leverage of one part of the body against another, for example, the chin against the neck to adjust the position of the vertebrae at the base of the skull. Cranial osteopathy tries to make minute adjustments to the bones of the skull by delicately manipulating the bones of the cranium and spine. Cranial osteopathy may be used to treat the same conditions as osteopathy itself. Osteopathy can claim many well-documented cures and is rapidly gaining acceptance by the medical profession. Before you have any osteopathic treatment, you should request X rays to exclude the possibility that you have osteoporosis (see p. 28).

CHIROPRACTIC

Chiropractic focuses on the anatomy of the spinal cord and on the nerves that branch out from it. Nerves run through each vertebra to the skin, bone, muscles, blood vessels, and organs. The theory is that manipulating a particular vertebra will influence the health of a certain organ. For example, because the liver is supplied by nerves from the middle thoracic (chest) vertebrae, manipulating them will affect liver function. Even

PRACTICING YOGA

Follow the guidelines below to make the most of this therapy.

• *Breathe deeply and rhythmically through your nose.*

• *Don't force yourself into a difficult position – some yoga positions can feel very uncomfortable at first.*

• *Work slowly toward becoming supple.*

• *Hold a posture only for as long as it is comfortable. Aim for about 30 seconds initially in standing and sitting postures.*

• *Wear comfortable, loose clothing and keep your feet bare to keep from slipping.*

• *Don't practice yoga for at least four hours after eating a large meal.*

relatively minor deviations of the anatomy of the spinal cord caused by conditions such as bad posture or inflammation, for instance, can impair the working of a nerve and the body part it supplies.

Vertebrae are manipulated using short, sharp thrusts designed to spring a bone back into place. This procedure demands great precision in placing the adjusting hand, and timing and directing the thrust.

Symptoms that respond best to chiropractic techniques are neck, muscle, shoulder, and joint pain. As with osteopathy, chiropractic should be used with caution on any menopausal women who might be suffering from osteoporosis (see p. 28) or who exhibit any signs of having very low bone mass.

YOGA

This is probably the best known of all the meditation and movement therapies. Its holistic approach, encompassing stretching movements, mental relaxation, and deep breathing, can help you deal very effectively with menopausal symptoms.

The aim of yoga postures, called *asanas*, is to encourage a healthy mind to exist in a healthy body and bring both into harmony. You can take up yoga whatever your age: you simply do as much as you find comfortable. Many people find that it helps them to overcome specific health problems, such as smoking or excessive drinking, high blood pressure, and menstrual problems.

Yoga must be learned slowly, avoiding all strain. It is simple and inexpensive to do – no equipment is needed, except perhaps a mat, a quiet room, and loose, comfortable clothing. You may find it easiest to have some training to start with to help you master the breathing techniques. *Asanas* seem to be a static way of conditioning the body. If you achieve the correct posture, however, each limb and muscle is stretching. After a series of *asanas*, allow yourself a period of relaxation in order to discipline and focus the mind, and create a calm mood before you resume your daily tasks.

It is generally felt that yoga promotes good posture and mental tranquility that may alleviate backache, mild depression, and sleeping problems. Consult your doctor before taking up yoga, however, if you suffer from any existing medical condition.

6

SEXUALITY AND RELATIONSHIPS

If you had an enjoyable and fulfilling sex life before menopause, you almost certainly will continue to have one afterward. In fact, there are many advantages to postmenopausal sex, one important one being that you no longer have to worry about contraception and pregnancy. Understanding the changes that are taking place in both your and your partner's body will help to maintain and enhance your sex life together. Following the simple guidance and suggestions in this chapter will enable you to continue enjoying a fulfilling physical relationship with your partner for the rest of your life.

Try the following suggestions for good vaginal health.

• *Apply yogurt containing live bacteria,* Lactobacillus acidophilus, *to the vagina. There is anecdotal evidence that it helps prevent infections. The yogurt should remain in the vagina for at least two hours after application – wearing a tampon can keep it from leaking out.*

• *Douche with a solution of one tablespoon of white vinegar in a pint of water. This will keep the vagina acidic. (Too much sugar in your urine can make your vagina alkaline and prone to infections, such as thrush.)*

• *Add a cup of vinegar to bath water or use a tampon soaked in the solution.*

• *Consult a qualified herbalist for herbal remedies – there are many available.*

If any treatment causes soreness, stop using it immediately.

NATURAL SATISFACTION

One benefit of growing older with a partner is that you know how to strike a balance between shared interests and privacy. A well-kept secret is that many of us lose our inhibitions as we get older. We feel free to enjoy sexual pleasure, to express ourselves in ways that we kept hidden when we were younger.

The saying "if you don't use it, you lose it" is particularly applicable to sex during menopause. Regular sexual activity can keep your sex organs healthy, and if you take care of yourself, you can remain sexually active for the rest of your life. There are, however, changes in your body, and often in your partner's body, that require adjustments to your familiar sexual routine. Once you know about these changes, you can begin to adapt your life accordingly to keep sex satisfying.

Factors that help sex after menopause
• A rewarding relationship before menopause.
• Positive attitudes toward sex and aging.
• A good relationship with your partner.
• Physical and emotional fitness, and an accepting attitude toward your body.

Factors that inhibit sex after menopause
• A history of unsatisfying sex.
• An unsupportive partner or an unhappy relationship.
• Problems such as vaginal dryness or soreness.
• Attitudes that equate sex with youthfulness or having children.
• Surgical removal of the ovaries.

VAGINAL CHANGES

During and after menopause, the walls of the vagina become drier and less elastic. Even the shape changes – it becomes shorter and narrower (although it always remains big enough to accommodate an erect penis). The clitoris becomes slightly smaller, and the lips of the vagina become thinner and flatter. The covering of the clitoris may also become thinner and pull back, leaving it more exposed. This can make it extremely sensitive to touch, and you may find that you need quite a bit of lubrication before it can be stimulated with the fingers.

In young women, one of the first signs of arousal is the wetness produced by the walls of the vagina. Droplets of fluid form a slippery coat in the vagina and on the vulva, making penetration easy and pleasurable for both partners. Falling estrogen levels mean that vaginal cells may not be able to lubricate as quickly as before. You may feel very aroused but it takes several minutes for your vagina to "catch up." If this is the case, explain to your partner that you need to take things slowly, and spend more time on foreplay.

In young women, thick vaginal walls serve as a cushion during intercourse, protecting both the bladder and the urethra from friction. At menopause, vaginal walls become thinner, and it is quite common to feel a strong urge to urinate after sex. If this is the case, empty your bladder promptly. Some menopausal women also complain of a burning sensation during urination that can persist for several days. Drinking plenty of water can relieve this feeling.

Although vaginal dryness is common during menopause, a small number of women still lubricate rapidly when aroused. The likely reason for this is that these women continue to have sex once or twice a week throughout their adult lives. This supports the belief that regular sex can promote vaginal health.

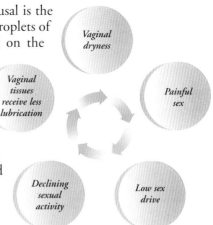

The vicious circle of vaginal dryness
The vagina and vulva become thin and prone to dryness after menopause, and this can make sex painful. Ironically, if you abstain from sex, the problem may get worse.

HORMONAL CHANGES

Sex drive is hormonally related, and many studies have shown that women experience heightened sexual desire around the middle of the menstrual cycle, which is the time when they usually ovulate.

Estrogen levels reach their peak at ovulation. However, ovulation is also marked by high levels of the male sex hormones, testosterone and androstenedione, and high levels of testosterone are known to create a high sex drive in both men and women. After menopause, the ratio of testosterone to estrogen becomes greater because estrogen levels fall while testosterone remains the same (or increases). Contrary to the myth of sexual decline, some women – about one in six – report increased sexual desire after menopause, which may be attributable to the relative excess of male hormones.

Research carried out on women who had undergone hysterectomies, including the removal of their ovaries, confirmed the role of testosterone in sexual arousal. The women were asked to rate the intensity of their sexual desire before and after their operations, and after surgery the women were given one of the following treatments: estrogen; testosterone; estrogen and testosterone; or a placebo. The study's conclusions were that only in those women taking testosterone or a mixture of estrogen and testosterone was sexual interest restored to pre-menopausal levels, and that male sex hormones do therefore stimulate women's sexual interest.

For this reason, the quantity of testosterone your menopausal ovaries produce is likely to have a significant effect on your sex drive. Hormone levels vary considerably from woman to woman: in some, blood levels of male hormones actually increase after menopause; in others, they decrease by 50 percent or more.

If you've noticed a decrease in sexual desire that seems to coincide with menopause – particularly if you have had a hysterectomy with your ovaries removed – it could be due to decreased levels of male sex hormones. Even if testosterone replacement therapy would seem to be an answer, it is not; there are two major problems. First, the ideal level of testosterone for women has not been determined, and doctors can only use blood tests as a guideline to determine how your level compares with what is normal for your age. Second, male sex hormones have potent side effects and can cause lowering of the voice and hirsutism (hairiness) to occur.

Rather than agree to use a therapy whose benefits can be mixed, therefore, it makes more sense to concentrate on simple, natural measures to sustain your interest in sex and in your partner. Kegel exercises (see p. 14) and the suggestions on p. 18 could both be helpful.

CHANGES IN YOUR PARTNER

An interested partner is the most important factor for good sex at any age, and the influence of declining hormones on desire may have a modest effect in comparison to the importance of a fulfilling relationship. Menopausal women usually have partners who are experiencing changes in their own sexual behavior, so it's helpful to be aware of male physiology, particularly if you have a partner over 50.

Changes in your partner's sexual behavior are easier to understand if you realize that there are changes in his hormones. As men age, testosterone-inhibiting factors increase, causing a decline in the frequency of erection. Replacing hormones in men is not as beneficial as it is in women. Men need a minimum amount of testosterone, and if they already have it, testosterone replacement therapy will not usually help.

Most young men can have an erection within seconds of being stimulated. For men over 50, it may take longer, and more direct stimulation of the penis may well be necessary. Some men find that they cannot maintain their erections for as long as they used to. This is not a problem, it just means that you have to adjust your timing where sex is concerned, so that you are fully aroused at the same time that he is ready for penetration. Mutual masturbation as part of foreplay can be helpful.

As a man ages, his penis becomes flaccid faster, and it may take longer for him to have another erection. For a man over 50, the waiting period may be 12 hours; for men in their 60s and 70s, it can take several days. Older men don't necessarily ejaculate during sex. If your partner doesn't ejaculate on one occasion, it doesn't mean that he will never ejaculate again. Each man is different and follows his own timetable.

There is a popular fallacy that aging robs a man of his capacity for sexual pleasure. It is not true, but many men are anxious about their sexual performance deteriorating. If your partner does not achieve an erection on more than one occasion, he may be afraid he is impotent and start avoiding sex altogether. This can lead to all sorts of misunderstandings: he may blame you, and you may feel guilty, or he may blame himself. It is therefore essential that you communicate frankly about your feelings.

SEEKING MEDICAL HELP

If your partner has severe problems getting or maintaining an erection, he should seek medical advice. Difficulties may well be physical in origin, particularly if he is taking certain medications. For instance, betablockers, which can be prescribed for high blood pressure, can affect sexual function, and so can antihistamines. In addition, diabetes can cause damage to the nerves that stimulate erection and ejaculation.

MAXIMIZE LOVEMAKING

One of the most important things you can do to nurture your sex life is to make the time to create a relaxing, sensual environment. Pay attention to mood and atmosphere, have a drink together, play your favorite music, and take turns at undressing each other. Using fragrant massage oil, gently stroke your partner all over, working your way slowly down his body from his head to his toes. When it's your turn, show your pleasure at what feels good, and be explicit about your preferences. Slowly move onto touching your partner's penis, and when he touches you, tell him what you would like him to do.

EVALUATING YOUR SEX LIFE

Take stock of your sex life by answering the following questions, which should help you assess your sex life and identify any areas that you would like to change. It may be useful for you and your partner to answer the questions together.

Your body
• Are you happy with your body?
• If you're not, are you prepared to improve your body by changing your diet and by exercising more?
• Are you inhibited about any one part of your body?
• Do you feel relaxed about undressing and being naked in front of your partner?

Your feelings
• Do you feel close to your partner?
• Do you think you and your partner are well matched sexually?
• Do you find it easy to talk about sex?
• Can you ask for what you want sexually?

The setting
• Where do you make love?
• Do you ever try to create a sexy atmosphere with soft lights, candles, or mood music?
• Do you always make love in the same place?
• Do you have complete privacy?

The buildup to sex
• How do you initiate sex?
• Do you give conflicting signals?
• If your partner misunderstands you, how can you communicate better?
• Do you spend enough time on foreplay so that you are fully aroused when you have sex?

Intercourse
• Do you ever find penetration difficult or painful?
• What do you do to overcome this?
• Do you reach orgasm and, if so, how?
• If you don't reach orgasm during intercourse, do you ask your partner to stimulate you in other ways?

Answering all of these questions could give you a better idea of what, if anything, you might want to change or improve about your sex life. For example, you may feel that making love has become routine and predictable. Suggestions about how to inject variety into your lovemaking are given in the pages that follow.

Genital touching can progress to penetration or can bring you both to orgasm. If you choose mutual masturbation, lubricate your hands with oil or a water-based jelly (don't use fragrant massage oil if you are going to use a condom because it destroys the rubber). Although some women may be inhibited about giving or receiving oral sex, it is another good way to extend foreplay, or it can be used as an end in itself.

Some couples like to increase their arousal by sharing their sexual fantasies or by looking at erotic material. Arousal begins in the brain, and if you are mentally stimulated, genital stimulation will usually follow.

Don't assume that because you have been making love to your partner for years, you know everything about him sexually. The secret of satisfying sex is to keep communicating with each other, asking your partner what he wants, telling him what you like, and sharing your sexual thoughts, dreams, and fantasies. Break away from your normal sexual routine – make love in a new position, in a new place, at a different time.

SENSUAL MASSAGE

The power of touch and its importance in our lives never diminishes. Even in very old age, the importance of physical intimacy and touch is high – being hugged and petted is necessary for our physical and mental well-being. A massage is an excellent way to relax: you can explore your partner's erogenous zones and set the scene for sex. Use fragranced massage oil or cream to lubricate his skin – apply it to your hands first to make it warm, then follow the tips on the right. Pay attention to parts of the body that are usually neglected, such as the feet.

EXTENDED FOREPLAY

The main reason for extending foreplay is that you and your partner may have slower sexual responses than you once had. Build up to sex gradually by stroking each other gently, and prolong the moment when you touch your partner's genitals by massaging him with fragranced oil. Other possibilities include having a bath or shower together and exploring your partner's erogenous zones by lightly nibbling them. When you touch your partner's genitals, spend time caressing him slowly until you both feel completely ready and eager for penetration.

SENSUAL MASSAGING

Try the following simple steps to help maximize your sensual experiences.

● *Lay your partner face down, sit astride his buttocks, and run your fingertips lightly up and down his back.*

● *Progress to firmer strokes, using the thumbs, paying special attention to muscles between the shoulder blades and at the base of the neck.*

● *Roll him onto his back and massage his abdomen and chest. Use your fingertips to circle his nipples with light strokes.*

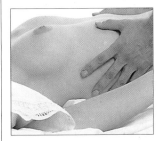

Erotic touching
Tell your partner where you'd like to be touched or demonstrate by guiding his hand.

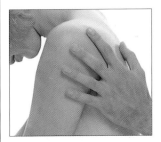

Sensual caresses
Spend time being stroked and caressed by your partner before you begin to make love.

MASTURBATING TECHNIQUES

If you have never masturbated, choose a time when you will be totally undisturbed and a place where you feel relaxed.

- *Start by stroking the whole of your body, then focus on your genital area. Some women stroke or press their entire vulva, others concentrate on stimulating the clitoral area.*

- *Stroke or rub with the fingers to provide intense stimulation; some women use a vibrator. Or climax by pressing your thighs together.*

- *Fantasizing may enhance arousal.*

Vibrators
You can use a vibrator to bring yourself to orgasm, or your partner can use it on you as a means of enhancing foreplay.

G-spot attachment

Standard variable-speed vibrator

Supple plastic vibrator

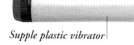

Control pad *Egg-shaped vibrator*

MASTURBATION
Self-stimulation is not only a safe form of sexual enjoyment, it is also an ideal way to explore your body and release sexual tension. If you don't have a partner, masturbation can provide vital sexual release – this can be a positive choice for many women. Even if you have a partner, you can use masturbation to complement intercourse. If you become aroused very slowly, your partner can spend time stimulating you manually. Alternatively, you can masturbate alone for pleasure. There are several different ways in which you can masturbate; see those listed on the left. Basically, however, whatever brings you satisfaction is absolutely fine, and you should never be afraid to experiment.

OVERCOMING PROBLEMS
Problems such as a low sex drive may be due to relationship problems or stress. Occasionally, there is a physiological basis, and you should always see a doctor to eliminate this possibility.

PROBLEMS ACHIEVING ERECTION
The first rule in achieving an erection is for your partner to learn to relax. Most sexual problems are psychological rather than physical in origin, and if your partner is anxious and afraid that he won't be able to achieve an erection, then he probably won't. If you feel your problems are particularly deep-rooted and that they are having a serious impact on your relationship, it may be useful to receive counseling.

Don't set out specifically to have intercourse, because this may put pressure on your partner. Spend a long time touching and stroking each other, and if he is aroused, concentrate on stimulating his genital area with your hands or mouth. If you use your hands to do this, lubricate the penis with a water-based jelly and massage the shaft firmly.

If your partner's problems result from medication he is taking, he should ask his doctor about alternatives. In severe cases of impotence, a penile implant consisting of two inflatable rods can be surgically installed in the penis. A pump in the scrotum inflates the rods, causing the penis to become erect.

LONG-TERM ILLNESS

Serious illness can be a major inhibiting factor in sex. This is particularly true if you or your partner have had heart problems. Because you are afraid of putting any extra pressure on your heart, you may abstain altogether. Fortunately, doctors agree that a normal sex life can greatly benefit people who have suffered heart attacks and other heart problems, and they encourage a return to normal sexual activity as soon as possible.

Arthritis can make intercourse uncomfortable, but pain can often be alleviated by some simple measures, such as having a hot bath to mobilize your joints, adopting a restful position during lovemaking, and taking painkilling medication an hour or so before having sex. The spoons position is gentle and relaxing. The woman lies on her side with her knee raised, while the man penetrates her from behind. This gives him access to her breasts and upper body, while she can stimulate herself manually. Always remember that sex does not have to be penetrative every time – alternatives such as oral sex, mutual masturbation, or stroking can also be stimulating.

Diabetes is another medical condition that can cause sexual problems. In women these include a dry, itchy vulva and yeast infections; in men they include difficulty in achieving an erection and problems ejaculating. Some diabetes medications can cause impotence, so check this with your doctor and ask about alternatives. If diabetes is treated early, all these problems may be lessened.

VAGINISMUS (VAGINAL SPASM)

Fear of penetration, which is sometimes referred to as vaginismus, can make sex very painful, and often impossible. The cause of vaginismus is almost always psychological and may stem from deep-rooted fears about sex. Some women develop it after menopause as a result of vaginal pain and dryness. They may become acutely sensitive to the stretching sensation that occurs during penetration and learn to anticipate pain, which triggers muscular contractions. If this is the case, there are effective self-help measures to alleviate postmenopausal sexual problems (see p. 18). If you had vaginismus before menopause, it may be a defensive reaction to sexual situations that you cannot control.

VAGINISMUS EXERCISES

Try the following simple techniques to ease penetration.

● *Using a mirror, touch the vaginal entrance with your fingers.*

● *Relax by breathing deeply, and when you feel ready, insert the tip of one finger into your vagina. Use a lubricant, such as oil, lubricating jelly, or saliva.*

● *Now insert your finger farther into the vagina – if you feel your vaginal muscles contracting, stop, wait until you feel relaxed, and try again. Using this technique, try to get to the point where you can insert two or three fingers into the vagina.*

● *When making love, experiment with woman-on-top positions, which allow you to control the depth of penetration.*

BIRTH CONTROL

Although menopause signals the end of fertility, women should continue to use birth control for at least one or two years after their last menstrual period. A common method of contraception chosen by women who have completed their families is the intrauterine device, or IUD, but other methods, such as oral contraceptives or condoms, are convenient and highly effective.

Spermicidal jelly
This is designed for use with a cap or a diaphragm. The jelly is squeezed into the diaphragm, which is then inserted into the vagina so that it covers the entrance to the cervix. Spermicidal creams and jellies are not effective contraceptives on their own.

Condoms are made from latex rubber or plastic

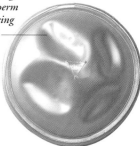

Contraceptive jelly containing vaginal spermicide

Male condom
This is the most widely used contraceptive in the world and it works by preventing sperm from entering the woman's body. It is rolled onto the erect penis before penetration and should be removed immediately after intercourse.

Triphasic pill

The diaphragm prevents sperm from entering the uterus

Mini-pill

Combination pill

Oral contraceptives
Combination pills contain estrogen and progestogen; triphasic pills contain three different doses of estrogen and progestogen; mini-pills contain progestogen only.

All brands of pills suppress ovulation

Diaphragm
The diaphragm is a soft rubber device with a flexible metal rim, designed to fit diagonally over the cervix. It is used with spermicidal jelly.

Intrauterine device (IUD)

This small plastic device is inserted into the uterus and can remain in place for several years. It works by preventing a fertilized egg from inplanting in the uterus.

The thread hangs down into the vagina

Vaginal sponge

This is impregnated with spermicide and should be put in water until it becomes foamy. It is then inserted deep into the vagina, where it will remain effective for up to 24 hours.

The sponge fits snugly over the cervix

Female condom

This is inserted into the vagina before sexual intercourse and removed immediately afterward. The open end of the female condom sits outside the body on the vulva.

The female condom is coated with spermicide for extra protection

TYPES OF CONTRACEPTION

TYPES	ADVANTAGES	DISADVANTAGES
Diaphragm and spermicide	The spermicide can act as a lubricant. Can be inserted before lovemaking and does not interfere with sex.	Difficult to see if you have a slight prolapse. May make urinary infections more likely, since the front rim of the diaphragm can press on the urethra.
Condoms (male and female)	Widely available without prescription. Protects against sexually transmitted diseases such as the HIV virus.	Effectiveness is lower than that of the pill or IUD. Condoms may sometimes interfere with a man's erection as he gets older.
Vaginal sponge	Easily available and can be self-fitted before intercourse.	Has the highest failure rate of all barrier contraceptives.
IUD	Very effective as a contraceptive. After insertion you can forget about it.	Requires insertion by a doctor. Some IUDs have to be removed due to irregular bleeding or infection.
Combined pill	High success rate. Offers protection against the risk of endometrial and ovarian cancer.	Carries more risk than barrier methods, e.g. thrombosis. Disguises menopause by regulating menstrual periods.
Progestogen only mini-pill	Suitable if you are advised not to take estrogen.	Has a slightly higher failure rate than the combined pill.

POSTMENOPAUSAL RELATIONSHIPS

Retirement can put a strain on marriages. Couples who live together quite happily in the evenings and on weekends find it can be hard to tolerate each other all the time. You might encounter problems that you never anticipated. Your partner might compensate for his loss of power at work by demanding excessive attention, and you might respond by nagging. The suggestions that follow may help alleviate stressful situations.

• Plan separate, as well as joint, activities.

• Try to arrange your home so that each of you has a room to escape to.

• Respect each other's friends, conversations, interests, and routines.

• Develop a common interest, such as a shared hobby, a small business venture, or an evening class.

• Keep talking to each other. Your partner can be your closest friend.

• Maintain a wide circle of friends; you'll need to plan not only for today but for the future, when one of you may be alone.

• Plan your finances together.

If a marriage has never been good and problems have never been resolved, the situation will be dramatically intensified when two people are thrown together for most of the time. Emotional strain at this time can be great, but preventable, if you tackle problems early on.

A full life includes physical love. If the frequency with which you and your partner make love declines, try to examine the reasons why. Some people believe that sex is dirty, indecent, or, at the very least, esthetically undesirable for older people. This attitude may spring from the traditional religious belief that sex for enjoyment only is wrong. These days, however, intercourse takes place more often for pleasure than for procreation. We know from many recent surveys that people in their 70s and beyond need and, indeed, have active sex lives. Sadly, this is often kept secret. We must realize that, as we become older, we still have the same capacity for physical love as we did 20 or 30 years ago, and this is the ideal time to cast aside taboos and inhibitions.

Many older couples find that sex is better in the morning, when they are refreshed, than in the evening, when they are more likely to be tired. In fact, a man's highest sexual hormone level occurs between four o'clock in the morning and noon, and his lowest around eight o'clock in the evening.

Masturbation should be encouraged, particularly for single women and women whose partners are infirm. No matter how frequently it is practiced, masturbation has no harmful effects.

DIVORCE

Marriage breakup gets harder as people get older. In the aftermath of divorce, many women fear that no one will desire them again. Some dislike going alone to social events after years of being accompanied by a partner, and some are bitter because they are left alone after 20 or more years of marriage. Financially, women may be very dependent on alimony, particularly if they haven't been trained for a job.

Pessimism can lead women to believe that divorce is the end of their lives. But having lived through the despair, pain, self-pity, and even self-hatred, many find that life improves. Some women get their first full-time job; others feel self-confident enough to go out with other men; yet others even enjoy sex for the first time in years after leaving a claustrophobic marriage, and find fulfillment with a new, more sympathetic partner.

If you go through a divorce in midlife, remember that there are many years ahead in which to enjoy yourself. If you are postmenopausal, you don't have to worry about getting pregnant, and if you have children, they are likely to be grown up and able to take care of themselves. Your biggest concern should be how best to maximize the potential of the years ahead.

SINGLE LIFE

If you are on your own, you have a variety of lifestyles open to you. You can live alone, sublet a room of your house, rent an apartment, or rent your home to tenants. You could even set up a commune: some 60-year-olds in Florida have gathered together and live in four homes as families, paying a younger couple to manage the homes and do the domestic work.

INDEX

A

acupressure, 77
acupuncture, 12, 29, 76
agnus castus, 13, 75–76
alcohol, controlling intake, 64–65
allopathy, 72
angina, 23
anxiety, 16, 24, 50, 52
aphrodisiacs, 18
appearance, importance of, 44–46
aromatherapy, 16, 73
arthritis, 69, 89

B

bad breath, 67
bad habits, abandoning, 64–65
birth control, 90–91
black cohosh, 12, 16, 76
bloating, 17, 20, 76
blood pressure, controlling, 31, 70
body, caring for, 36–37, 66–70
body mass, 28
body shape, and heart disease, 24
bone density tests, 28, 29
bowel symptoms, 20
breast cancer, 34
breast symptoms, 21
breathing techniques, 43
breathlessness, 70
brittle bones disease, 15
see also osteoporosis

C

caffeine, reducing intake, 65
calcium absorption, 48, 49, 51
calcium-rich foods, 15, 29, 48
chilblains, 69
chiropractic, 79–80
cholesterol levels, lowering, 23
climacteric, 8–9
clothes, choosing, 44–45
collagen deficiency, 15, 16, 49
colonic irrigation, 20

complementary medicine, 72–80
see also herbal remedies
concentration, lack of 26
constipation, 20
contraception, 90–91
cystitis, 14, 32

D

depression, 13, 24–25
alleviating, 25–26, 50, 52, 73
diabetes, 50, 52, 89
diet:
bad foods, 54–55
balanced, 13, 19, 56–57
healthy, 48, 51
diuretics, 54, 64
diverticulitis, 20, 53
divorce, 93
dribbling urine, 14
drinking, healthy, 14, 17, 50
see also abandoning bad habits

E

ear wax, 67
emotional symptoms, 24–26
essential oils, 15, 16, 73
estrogen:
and digestion, 20
lowered levels, 17, 22, 28, 50, 83
topping up with exercise, 58
exercise, benefits of, 23–24, 58–59
exercises, body, 60–63
yoga, 80
eyes, and collagen deficiency, 16
eyesight, deterioration in, 66

F, G

face symptoms, 17
family roles, changing, 38–39
fat intake, 48, 54–55
fatigue, 15, 16
alleviating, 50, 52, 73
feet, caring for, 68–69
fiber, importance of, 53
fit, keeping, 58–63

foods, bad, 54–55
foreplay, extended, 87–88
forgetfulness, 26
formication, 17
fractures, bone, 28
genitals, caring for, 67–68
grandparent, role as, 38–39
gums, 16, 67

H

hair, and collagen deficiency, 16
hair care, 46
halitosis, 67
hearing loss, 66
heart attacks, 30–31
heart symptoms, 23–24
herbal remedies:
aphrodisiacs, 18
breast pains, 21
depression, 25
hot flashes, 12, 75
muscle and joint symptoms, 15
night sweats, 13
PMS, 16
purgatives, 20
sleep-inducing, 19
urinary symptoms, 14
herbalism, 75–76
high-stress foods, 55
homeopathy, 74
hormonal changes, 83–84
hormone replacement therapy (HRT), 49
hot flashes, 11, 64
alleviating, 12, 50, 52, 75
hydrotherapy, 77
hypertension, 23, 52
hypothyroidism, 18–19, 22–23, 50, 52

I

impotence, 18
incontinence, 14, 33
insomnia, 12, 13, 16
intellectual deterioration, 26, 70
irritability, 16, 24, 42, 52
irritable bowel syndrome, 53
itchiness, 17, 32–33

J, K, L

joint symptoms, 15
Kegel exercises, 14, 19, 33, 84
kidneys, looking after, 70
legs, caring for, 68–69
lovemaking, maximizing,
    86–89, 92–93
lungs, effects of aging, 70

M

massage, 77–79
    neuromuscular, 78–79
    sensual, 87
    Swedish, 78
    using essential oils, 73
mastalgia, 21
masturbation, 88, 93
medicines, and diminishing
    sexual desire, 18
meditation, 13, 42–43
memory maintenance, 41
menopause:
    average age experienced, 9
    precise meaning, 9
    symptoms, 10–26
    timetable, 8–9
menstrual bleeding, excessive,
    50, 52
mental fitness, 40–41, 58–59
mental relaxation, deep,
    42–43
mind, taking control of, 37
mineral depleters, 54
minerals, beneficial, 51–53
mood swings, 16, 25, 50
mouth, 16, 17, 67
muscle relaxation, deep, 42
muscle symptoms, 15

N, O

nails, 16, 69
natural therapies, 72–80
naturopathy, 72
night sweats, 12–13, 74
nutrient depleters, 54
nutrition, good, 48–55
osteopathy, 79
osteoporosis, 15, 28–29, 48, 64
    preventing, 29, 49, 50, 52

P

palpitations, 11
parents, caring for, 38
partner, sexual changes, 84–85,
    88
penetration, fear of, 89
perimenopause, 9
period, age of last, 9
positive thinking, 36–37
postmenopause, 9
posture, good, 44
premenopause, 8
premenstrual symptoms,
    16–17
premenstrual syndrome
    (PMS), 16, 74
progesterone, 20, 26
pruritis vulvae, 32–33
purgatives, 20

R, S

relationships, postmenopausal,
    92–93
relaxation, 13, 42–43
sage tea, preparing, 75
salt, reducing intake, 55
self-esteem, maintaining, 37, 44
sex, postmenopausal, 17–19,
    82–89, 92–93
shoes, choosing, 45, 68
single life, 93
skin symptoms, 16, 17, 69
sleeplessness, 12, 13, 16
smoking, controlling, 11, 64
stomach symptoms, 20
stress, 19, 40, 42
    reducing, 42–43
strokes, 30–31
sugar, reducing intake, 54
sun, exposure to, 17

T, U, V

teeth, caring for, 67
temperature, body, 11
testosterone, 83–84
urinary symptoms, 14
urogenital aging, 32–33
vaginal dryness, 14, 18, 82–83
    relieving, 51, 74

vaginal health, 67–68, 82, 83
vaginismus, 89
varicose veins, 69
vibrators, 88
vitamin depleters, 54
vitamins, beneficial, 49–51
voice, lowering of, 22–23

W, Y, Z

waist-to-hip ratios, 24
water, importance of, 53–54
water retention, 16, 17
water treatments, 77
weight control, 22, 56–57
wrinkles, facial, 17
yoga, 13, 80
zinc-rich foods, 19

ACKNOWLEDGMENTS

The publisher would like to thank the following
individuals and organizations for their
contribution to this book.

ADDITIONAL EDITORIAL ASSISTANCE
Nicky Adamson, Maureen Rissik,
Constance M. Robinson

PHOTOGRAPHY
Jules Selmes, Steve Head (assistant)

ILLUSTRATION
Tony Graham, Sue Sharples, Joanna Cameron,
Joe Lawrence, Howard Pemberton, Coral Mula

PAPER SCULPTOR
Clive Stephens

EXERCISES
Juliette Kando devised and performed the
movements on pp. 60–61/pp. 62–63
Kando Studios, 88 Victoria Road
London NW6 6QA

EQUIPMENT
Ann Summers, Boots, Braun UK, Colourings by
The Body Shop, Kays Shoes, Marie Stopes Clinic,
Neal's Yard Remedies, Rigby and Peller,
St. Bartholomew's Hospital

INDEX
Robert Hood

TEXT FILM
The Brightside Partnership, London